Contents

Detailed contents

Preventive Cardiology: A Practical Manual

C.S. Jennings
Cardiovascular Specialist Research Nurse
Cardiovascular Medicine, National Heart and Lung Institute, Imperial College London

A.C. Mead
Specialist Dietitian
Imperial College Healthcare NHS Trust and National Heart and Lung Institute, Imperial College London

J.L. Jones
Specialist Physiotherapist
Cardiovascular Medicine, National Heart and Lung Institute, Imperial College London

A.M. Holden
Physical Activity Specialist
Cardiovascular Medicine, National Heart and Lung Institute, Imperial College London

S.B. Connolly
Consultant Cardiologist, Imperial College Healthcare NHS Trust
Honorary Senior Lecturer, National Heart and Lung Institute, Imperial College London

K.P. Kotseva
Consultant Cardiologist
Imperial College Healthcare NHS Trust, Senior Clinical Research Fellow, Cardiovascular Medicine, National Heart and Lung Institute, Imperial College London

and D.A. Wood
Garfield Weston Chair of Cardiovascular Medicine
National Heart and Lung Institute, Imperial College London

OXFORD
UNIVERSITY PRESS

OXFORD
UNIVERSITY PRESS

Great Clarendon Street, Oxford OX2 6DP

Oxford University Press is a department of the University of Oxford.
It furthers the University's objective of excellence in research, scholarship,
and education by publishing worldwide in

Oxford New York

Auckland Cape Town Dar es Salaam Hong Kong Karachi
Kuala Lumpur Madrid Melbourne Mexico City Nairobi
New Delhi Shanghai Taipei Toronto

With offices in

Argentina Austria Brazil Chile Czech Republic France Greece
Guatemala Hungary Italy Japan Poland Portugal Singapore
South Korea Switzerland Thailand Turkey Ukraine Vietnam

Oxford is a registered trade mark of Oxford University Press
in the UK and in certain other countries

Published in the United States
by Oxford University Press Inc., New York

First published 2009

British Library Cataloguing in Publication Data
Data available

Library of Congress Cataloging in Publication Data
Data available

Typeset by Cepha Imaging Private Ltd., Bangalore, India
Printed in Italy
on acid-free paper by
Lego S. p. A.

ISBN 978–0–19–923630–5

10 9 8 7 6 5 4 3 2 1

Oxford University Press makes no representation, express or implied, that the drug dosages in this book are correct. Readers must therefore always check the product information and clinical procedures with the most up to date published product information and data sheets provided by the manufacturers and the most recent codes of conduct and safety regulations. The authors and publishers do not accept responsibility or legal liability for any errors in the text or for the misuse or misapplication of material in this work.

Foreword

Modern cardiovascular medicine has witnessed a transformation in the acute management of vascular patients, giving more years to life. However, salvaging the acutely ischaemic myocardium by primary angioplasty for example is important but already too late in the management of coronary patients. We need to address the underlying causes of the disease which precipitated the acute event in order to reduce the risk of recurrent disease.

The watch word is *prevention*. All patients with vascular disease should be able to access a comprehensive preventive cardiology programme addressing lifestyle, risk factor management, and cardioprotective drugs. The multi-disciplinary team - nurses, dietitians, physiotherapists, physical activity specialists, occupational therapists, psychologists, pharmacists and others – need to work together with cardiologists and GPs to deliver such preventive care.

This Care Manual in Preventive Cardiology serves the professional interests of all members of the team by giving practical advice on every aspect of prevention. Waiting until patients develop vascular disease will be too late for some and the preventive cardiology team should extend their services to those people who are at high risk of developing cardiovascular disease in the community. Prevention is always better than cure.

Professor Kim Fox

Preface

The European and British guidelines on cardiovascular disease prevention in clinical practice[1,2] advocate that the care of all high-risk patients and their families should embrace all aspects of cardiovascular prevention and rehabilitation. High-risk patients are those who present with symptomatic atherosclerotic disease and those who are asymptomatic but at high total risk of developing atherosclerotic disease (see figure below). If prevention initiatives are to have the greatest impact and be cost effective, they should be targeted at these high-risk patients and their families.

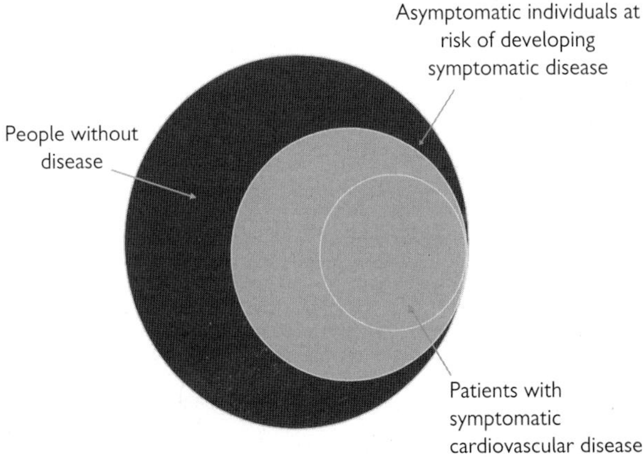

High-risk patients and their families require multidisciplinary support to achieve appropriate lifestyle change—quitting smoking, making healthier food choices, and increasing physical activity—based on behavioural models of change. Risk factor management in terms of controlling weight, blood pressure, lipids and glucose and the use of prophylactic drug therapies, such as aspirin, beta-blockers, angiotensin-converting enzyme (ACE) inhibitors, lipid modification therapy, and anticoagulants, is also an integral part of this approach. The traditional focus of cardiac rehabilitation on physical rehabilitation for coronary disease is gradually evolving into a more comprehensive strategy for all atherosclerotic disease patients which addresses all aspects of lifestyle, the management of other risk factors and the use of cardioprotective drug therapies.

Beyond those with established cardiovascular disease, the next challenge is to reach those apparently healthy individuals who are at high risk of developing cardiovascular disease. Both the European and the British guidelines on cardiovascular disease prevention provide models for total risk estimation (see risk estimation charts in this manual).

Total cardiovascular risk is estimated from the major risk factors: age, gender, smoking, total cholesterol (or the ratio of total to high-density lipoprotein (HDL) cholesterol), and blood pressure. Total cardiovascular risk means integrating the contribution of all these risk factors to estimate the probability (chance) of a major cardiovascular event over the next 10 years. In addition, other co-morbidities, such as overweight and central obesity, a sedentary lifestyle, a family history of premature cardiovascular disease (CVD), triglycerides, and diabetes have to be taken into account. Identification of high-risk individuals for a preventive cardiology programme should therefore be based on this concept of total cardiovascular risk and not on single risk factors.

This holistic approach presents a major challenge to health professionals, who are accustomed to working within their specialties of cardiac rehabilitation, hypertension, dyslipidaemia, and diabetes, to join forces in an integrated coalition in order to provide comprehensive care for all of these high-risk patients and their families.

This preventive cardiology care manual has been written by a multidisciplinary team for the multidisciplinary team. It provides a comprehensive approach to preventive cardiology care for all high-risk patients and their families. Our manual is directed at doctors, nurses, dietitians, and physiotherapists or other physical activity specialists. It provides a guide to these professionals on how to manage high-risk patients and their families through a preventive cardiology programme.

The manual takes the professional through the patient and family pathway—from patient identification, recruitment of patient and family, comprehensive assessment of lifestyle and cardiovascular risk factors, to management of lifestyle change, reduction of cardiovascular risk factors and compliance with cardioprotective drug therapies. The role of each member of the multidisciplinary team is described, together with the tools available to achieve lifestyle and risk-factor change.

This manual is based on the EUROACTION model of preventive cardiology care. EUROACTION was a European Society of Cardiology demonstration project in preventive cardiology. The principal results of this cluster randomized controlled trial are published in the *Lancet*.[3]

The manual covers:

- The rationale for our model of preventive cardiology care.
- Bringing together a core multidisciplinary team.
- Methods of identification of coronary patients and asymptomatic individuals at high risk of developing cardiovascular disease.
- Inclusion of families.
- Risk estimation using evidence-based nationally and internationally recognized tools.
- Conducting a family-based multidisciplinary assessment of lifestyle and other cardiovascular risk factors.
- Individualized goal setting for lifestyle.
- Principles of smoking cessation.
- Principles of a cardioprotective diet and managing dietary change.
- Principles of helping patients and families to become physically active.
- Principles of managing weight loss in the overweight and obese.
- Protocols for blood pressure, lipid, and glucose management.
- Prescription and titration of cardioprotective medications and compliance.

- Running a supervised exercise programme.
- Co-ordinating educational workshops.
- Following up first-degree relatives.
- Key references for evidence base, assessment tools, behavioural strategies, guidelines, and treatment protocols.

1 JBS2 (2005). Joint British Societies' guidelines on prevention of cardiovascular disease in clinical practice. *Heart*, **91**(Suppl 5), v1–v52.

2 Graham, I., Atar, D., Borch-Johnsen, K. *et al.* (2007). European guidelines on cardiovascular disease prevention in clinical practice: full text. Fourth Joint Task Force of the European Society of Cardiology and other Societies on Cardiovascular Disease Prevention in Clinical Practice. *European Journal of Cardiovascular Prevention and Rehabilitation*, **14**(Suppl 2), S1–S113.

3 Wood, D.A., Kotseva, K., Connolly, S. *et al.*, on behalf of EUROACTION Study Group. (2008). Nurse-coordinated multidisciplinary, family-based cardiovascular disease prevention programme (EUROACTION) for patients with coronary heart disease and asymptomatic individuals at high risk of cardiovascular disease: a paired, cluster-randomised controlled trial. *Lancet*, **371**, 1999–2012.

Summary of lifestyle, risk factor, and therapeutic targets

The role of the preventive cardiology multidisciplinary team is to help people with atherosclerotic cardiovascular disease, individuals at high risk of developing cardiovascular disease, and their families to achieve the following lifestyle, risk factor, and therapeutic goals.

- Not smoking.
- Eating a cardioprotective diet defined as:
  - Total intake of fat ≤30% of total energy intake.
  - Intake of saturated fats to ≤10% of total energy intake.
  - Intake of cholesterol <300 mg/day.
  - Replace saturated fats by an increased intake of unsaturated fats, particularly monounsaturated fat.
  - Increase intake of fresh fruit and vegetables to at least five portions per day.
  - Regular intake of fish and other sources of omega-3 fatty acids (at least two servings of fish per week). After myocardial infarction, patients should aim for 2–4 large portion of oily fish/week or take a supplement (1 g/d eicosapentaenoic acid and docosahexaenoic acid).
  - Limit alcohol intake to <21 units per week (men) and <14 units per week (women) or <3-4 units/day (men) and <2-3 units per day (women) with 2 alcohol free days per week.
  - Limit intake of salt to <100 mmol/l per day (<6 g of sodium chloride or <2.4 g of sodium per day).
- Becoming more physically active, defined as regular aerobic physical activity of at least 30 min/day, most days of the week (e.g. brisk walking/swimming).
- Achieving and maintaining a healthy shape and weight:
  - White Caucasians: waist circumference ***below*** 94 cm for men and ***below*** 80 cm for women; Asians: below 90 cm for men and below 80 cm for women.
  - Body mass index ***below*** 25 kg/m^2.
- Blood pressure ***below*** 140/85 mmHg (and for those with coronary disease and/or diabetes ***below*** 130/80 mmHg).
- Total cholesterol ***below*** 4 mmol/l (low-density lipoprotein cholesterol ***below*** 2 mmol/l) or a 25% reduction.
- Fasting plasma glucose ***below*** 6.1 mmol/l. HbA_{1c} < 6.5% in all persons with diabetes or impaired glucose regulation.
- To ensure that ***each*** of the following classes of cardioprotective medications is prescribed as clinically indicated***, at the doses used in the*** clinical trials, for coronary patients, individuals at high risk, and their families, and to encourage long-term compliance with these therapies:
  - anti-platelet therapy
  - beta-blockers

  - angiotensin-converting enzyme (ACE) inhibitors or A2 receptor blockers
  - other antihypertensive medications
  - lipid-lowering therapy (statins).
- Screening of first-degree relatives of people with premature atherosclerotic disease (men <55 years and women <65 years).

Abbreviations

AACVPR	American Association of Cardiovascular and Pulmonary Rehabilitation
ABV	alcohol by volume
ACE	angiotensin-converting enzyme
ACPICR	Association of Chartered Physiotherapists in Cardiac Rehabilitation
ACSM	American College of Sports Medicine
AF	Activity Factor
ALT	Alanine transaminase
AR	active recovery
ARB	Angiotensin receptor blocker
BACR	British Association for Cardiac Rehabilitation
BIA	bioelectrical impedance analysis
BMI	body mass index
BMR	basal metabolic rate
BP	blood pressure
bpm	beats per minute
CBT	cognitive behavioural therapy
CCU	Coronary Care Unit
CHD	coronary heart disease
CHF	congestive heart failure
CI	contraindication
COPD	chronic obstructive pulmonary disease
CR	category ratio
CT	computed tomography
CV	cardiovascular
CVD	cardiovascular disease
CVPR	cardiovascular disease prevention and rehabilitation programme
DHA	docosahexaenoic acid
ECG	electrocardiogram
ED	erectile dysfunction
EF	ejection fraction
ENRICHD1	Enhancing Recovery in Coronary Heart Disease Patients
EPA	eicosapentaenoic acid
ESSI	ENRICHD Social Support Instrument
ETT	exercise tolerance test

FITT	frequency, intensity, time, type
FTND	Fagerström Test for Nicotine Dependence
GI	glycaemic index
GMS	Global Mood Scale
GTN	glycerol trinitrate
HADS	Hospital Anxiety and Depression Scale
HbA1c	haemoglobin A1c
HDL	high-density lipoprotein
HDL-C	high-density lipoprotein cholesterol
HRmax	heart rate maximum
HRQoL	Health Related Quality of Life
HRR	heart rate reserve
IFG	impaired fasting glycaemia
IGT	impaired glucose tolerance
IIEF	International Index of Erectile Function
ILS	immediate life support
IPQ-R	Illness Perception Questionnaire
ITU	intensive care unit
IV	intravenous
JBS2	Joint British Societies' Second Guidelines on prevention of cardiovascular disease in clinical practice
JES4	Joint European Societies' Fourth Guidelines on cardiovascular disease prevention in clinical practice
LDL	low-density lipoprotein
LDL-C	low-density lipoprotein cholesterol
MET	metabolic equivalent
MI	myocardial infarction
MUFA	monounsaturated fatty acids
NACR	National Audit for Cardiac Rehabilitation
NRT	nicotine replacement therapy
NSTEMI	non-ST elevation myocardial infarction
NYHA	New York Heart Association
OGTT	oral glucose tolerance test
PA	physical activity
PAD	peripheral arterial disease
PCOS	polycystic ovary syndrome
PDE-5	phosphodiesterase type 5
PUFA	polyunsaturated fatty acids
QALYs	quality-adjusted life years
RPE	rating of perceived exertion
SFA	saturated fatty acids

SOB	shortness of breath
SSRI	selective serotonin reuptake inhibitor
STEMI	ST elevation myocardial infarction
TAG	triacylglycerols
TC	total cholesterol
TFA	trans fatty acids
TG	triglycerides
THRR	Training Heart Rate Range
TIA	transient ischaemic attack
WC	waist circumference
WHO	World Health Organization
WHR	waist hip ratio

Part 1

Background and multidisciplinary family-based cardiovascular assessment

Chapter 1

Rationale for preventive cardiology programmes

What is preventive cardiology?

The overall aim of preventive cardiology is to reduce the risk of developing symptomatic atherosclerotic disease among apparently healthy high-risk individuals in the general population. In those patients who do develop the disease and survive, the aim is to reduce their risk of recurrent cardiovascular disease (CVD) and death. Preventive cardiology therefore aims to improve both quality of life and life expectancy in people at increased risk of developing CVD and patients with established disease.

Priorities for CVD prevention

- People with any form of established atherosclerotic CVD.
- Asymptomatic people without established CVD but with risk factor combinations putting them at high total risk of developing atherosclerotic CVD.
- People with diabetes mellitus (type 1 or 2).
- Markedly elevated single risk factors with target organ damage.
- Familial dyslipidaemia, such as familial hypercholesterolaemia or familial combined hyperlipidaemia.
- People with a family history of premature CVD (men <55 years, women <65 years).

Objectives of CVD prevention (JES4)

- To assist people at low CVD risk to maintain this state thoughout life and to help those at higher CVD risk to reduce it.
- To achieve the characteristics of people who tend to stay healthy:
  - no smoking
  - healthy food choices
  - physical activity: 30 min of moderate activity/daily
  - body mass index (BMI) < 25 kg/m^2 and avoidance of central obesity
  - blood pressure (BP) < 140/90 mmHg in most
  - total cholesterol < 5 mmol/l (~190 mg/dl)
  - low-density lipoprotein (LDL) cholesterol < 3 mmol/l (~115 mg/dl)
  - blood glucose < 6 mmol/l (~110 mg/dl).
- To achieve more rigorous risk factor control in high-risk subjects, especially those with established CVD or diabetes:
  - BP < 130/80 mmHg
  - total cholesterol < 4.5 mmol/l (~175 mg/dl) with an option of <4 mmol/l (~155 mg/dl) if feasible
  - LDL cholesterol < 2.5 mmol/l (~100 mg/dl) with an option of <2 mmol/l (~80 mg/dl) if feasible
  - fasting blood glucose < 6 mmol/l (~110 mg/dl) and haemoglobin A1$_c$ (HbA1$_c$) < 6.5% if feasible.
- To consider cardioprotective drug therapy in high-risk patients and especially those with established atherosclerotic CVD.

Objectives of CVD prevention: lifestyle, risk-factor and therapeutic targets in high-risk people (JBS2)

- Lifestyle
  - no smoking
  - healthy food choices
  - physical activity: regular aerobic physical activity of at least 30 min per day, most days of the week.
- Other risk factors:
  - BMI < 25 kg/m^2 and avoidance of central obesity
  - BP < 140/85 mmHg in asymptomatic people at high risk
  - (<130/80 mmHg in people with atherosclerotic cardiovascular disease or diabetes)
  - total cholesterol < 4 mmol/l (~155 mg/dl) or a 25% reduction
  - LDL cholesterol < 2 mmol/l (~80 mg/dl) or a 30% reduction
  - blood glucose ≤ 6 mmol/l (~110 mg/dl) and $HbA1_c$ < 6.5%.
- To consider cardioprotective drug therapy in high-risk patients and especially those with established atherosclerotic CVD.

What is a high-risk patient?

- Patients with established atherosclerotic CVD, whether of the coronary, peripheral, cerebral vessels, or of the aorta, even if asymptomatic.
- Asymptomatic individuals who are at increased risk of CVD because of:
  - multiple risk factors resulting in raised total CVD risk:
    JES4:[1] total CVD risk (SCORE) ≥ 5% 10-year risk of CVD death
    JBS2:[2] total CVD risk ≥ 20% over 10 years of developing atherosclerotic CVD
  - diabetes type 2 and type 1
  - markedly increased single risk factors, especially if associated with end-organ damage:
    JES4: blood pressure ≥ 180/110 mmHg; total cholesterol ≥ 8 mmol/l (~320 mg/dl), LDL cholesterol ≥ 6 mmol/l (~240 mg/dl)
    JBS2: blood pressure ≥ 160/100 mmHg; total cholesterol/HDL cholesterol ratio ≥ 6.
- Close relatives of subjects with premature atherosclerotic CVD or of those at particularly high risk.

1 Graham, I., Atar, D., Borch-Johnsen, K. *et al.* (2007). European guidelines on cardiovascular disease prevention in clinical practice: full text. Fourth Joint Task Force of the European Society of Cardiology and other Societies on Cardiovascular Disease Prevention in Clinical Practice. *European Journal of Cardiovascular Prevention and Rehabilitation*, **14**(Suppl 2), S1–S113.

2 British Cardiac Society, British Hypertension Society, Diabetes UK, HEART UK, Primary Care Cardiovascular Society, The Stroke Association. JBS2 (2005) Joint British Societies' guidelines on prevention of cardiovascular disease in clinical practice. *Heart*, **91**(Suppl V), V1–V5.

Table 1.1 Lifestyle, physiological, biochemical and other characteristics associated with increased risk of cardiovascular disease

Lifestyle	Physiological or biochemical characteristics	Other characteristics
Diet high in saturated fat, cholesterol and calories	Elevated blood pressure	Age
Tobacco smoking	Elevated plasma total cholesterol (LDL-cholesterol)	Sex
Excess alcohol consumption	Low plasma HDL-cholesterol	Family history of coronary heart disease (CHD) or other atherosclerotic vascular disease at early age (in men <55 years, in women <65 years)
Physical inactivity	Elevated plasma triglycerides	Personal history of CHD or other atherosclerotic vascular disease
Obesity and central obesity	Elevated plasma glucose/ diabetes	
	Thrombogenic factors	

What is cardiovascular risk?

Absolute multifactorial risk

Absolute risk of CVD is the probability of an individual developing the disease over a defined period (e.g. within the next 10 years).

As CVD is multifactorial in its origins, it is important, in estimating the risk of developing or having recurrent CVD, to consider all risk factors simultaneously:

- The overall level of risk is based on all factors taken together.
- Physicians deal with the whole patient rather than one aspect of his or her risk.
- Clustering of risk factors in an individual may have a multiplicative effect on absolute disease risk.
- An individual with a number of mildly abnormal risk factors may be at greater absolute CVD risk than a subject with just one high risk factor.

Relative risk

Relative risk is the ratio of absolute CHD risk for an individual with one or more risk factors to that of an individual at a reference level of risk. Two different ways of defining the reference level of risk have been used:

- the absolute risk for a person at low risk (i.e. a person of the same age and sex, but without any major risk factors); and
- the absolute risk for a person of the same age and sex with average risk in the population.

Relative risk informs an individual of their risk in relation to that of their peers, and is particularly valuable in younger people who are always at low absolute risk.

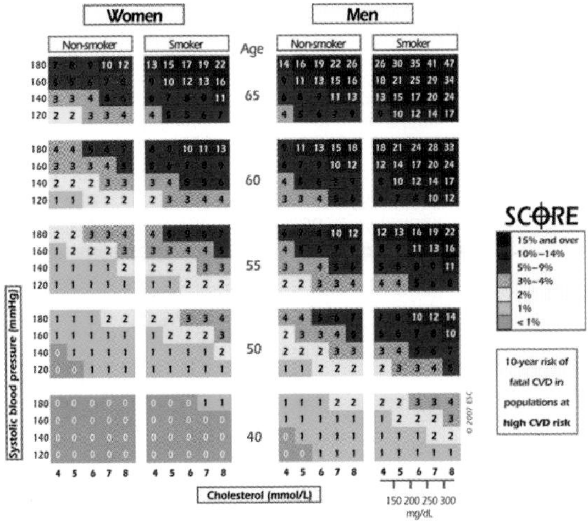

Plate 1 SCORE chart: 10-year risk of fatal CVD in populations at high CVD risk. Risk factors: age, gender, smoking, systolic blood pressure, and total cholesterol. Reproduced from the original version of the European Guidelines on CVD Prevention. Executive Summary (European Heart Journal 2007;28:2375-2414) and Full text (European Journal of Cardiovascular Prevention and Rehabilitation 2007;14(suppl 2):S1-S113). Reproduced with permission of the European Society of Cardiology. © 2007 ESC.

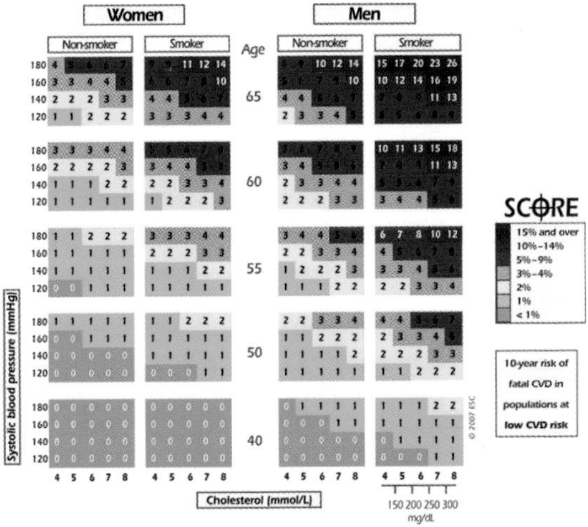

Plate 2 SCORE chart: 10-year risk of fatal CVD in populations at low CVD risk. Risk factors: age, gender, smoking, systolic blood pressure, and total cholesterol. Reproduced from the original version of the European Guidelines on CVD Prevention. Executive Summary (European Heart Journal 2007;28:2375-2414) and Full text (European Journal of Cardiovascular Prevention and Rehabilitation 2007;14(suppl 2):S1-S113). Reproduced with permission of the European Society of Cardiology. © 2007 ESC.

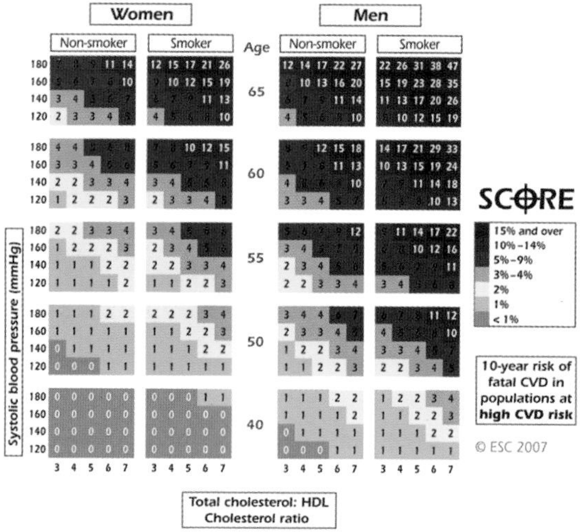

Plate 3 SCORE chart: 10-year risk of fatal CVD in populations at low CVD risk. Risk factors: age, gender, smoking, systolic blood pressure, and total cholesterol. Reproduced from the original version of the European Guidelines on CVD Prevention. Executive Summary (European Heart Journal 2007;28:2375-2414) and Full text (European Journal of Cardiovascular Prevention and Rehabilitation 2007;14(suppl 2):S1-S113). Reproduced with permission of the European Society of Cardiology. © 2007 ESC.

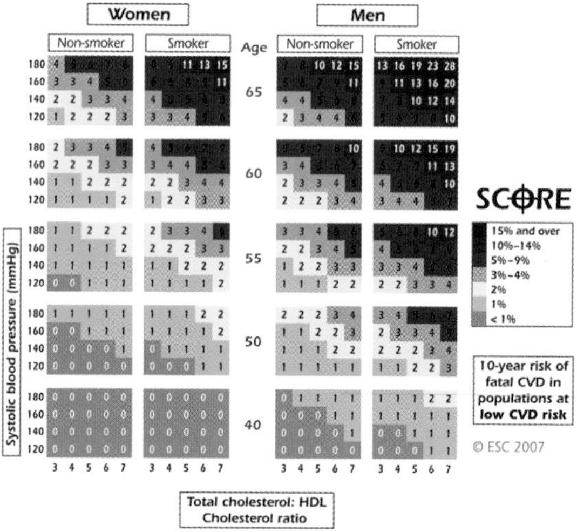

Plate 4 SCORE chart: 10-year risk of fatal CVD in populations at low CVD risk. Risk factors: age, gender, smoking, systolic blood pressure, and total cholesterol. Reproduced from the original version of the European Guidelines on CVD Prevention. Executive Summary (European Heart Journal 2007;28:2375-2414) and Full text (European Journal of Cardiovascular Prevention and Rehabilitation 2007;14(suppl 2):S1-S113). Reproduced with permission of the European Society of Cardiology. © 2007 ESC.

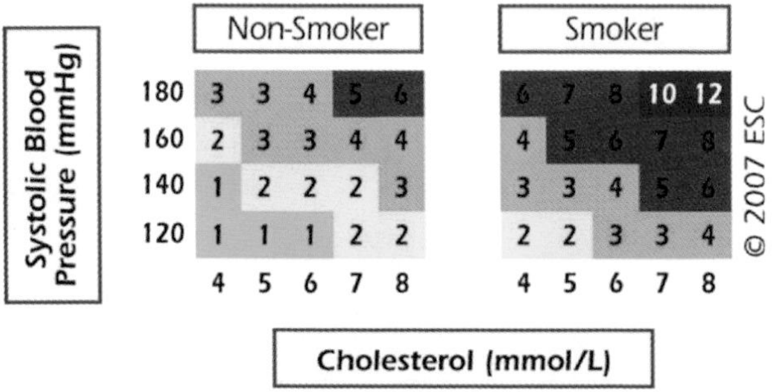

Plate 5 Relative risk chart. Reproduced from the original version of the European Guidelines on CVD Prevention. Executive Summary (European Heart Journal 2007;28:2375-2414) and Full text (European Journal) of Cardiovascular Prevention and Rehabilitation 2007;14 (suppl 2):S1-S113). Reproduction with permission of the European Society of Cardiology. © 2007 ESC. (see fig 1.1 p 11)

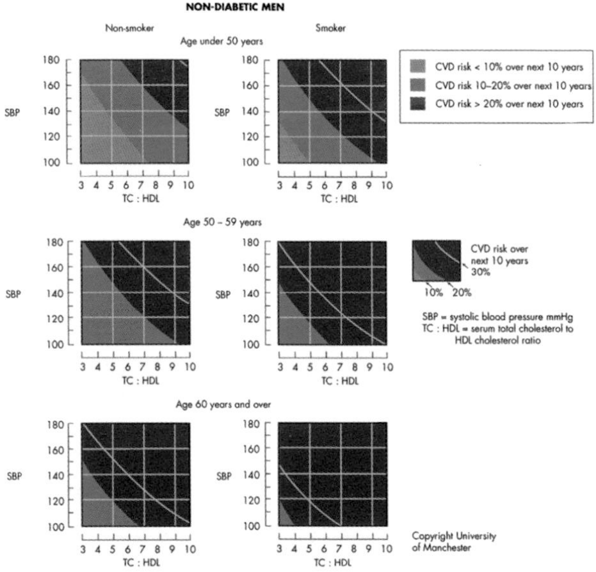

Plate 6 Joint British Societies' CVD risk prediction chart: non-diabetic men. (See fig 1.2 p 14)

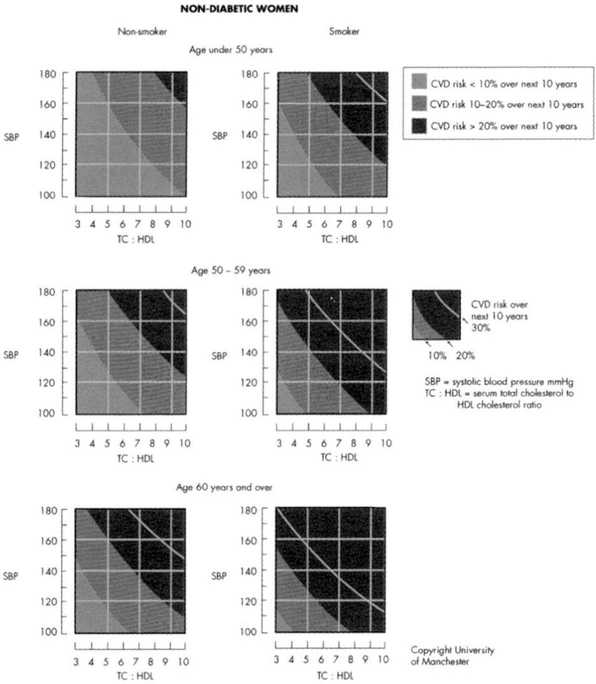

Plate 7 Joint British Societies' CVD risk prediction chart: non-diabetic women. (See fig 1.3 p 15)

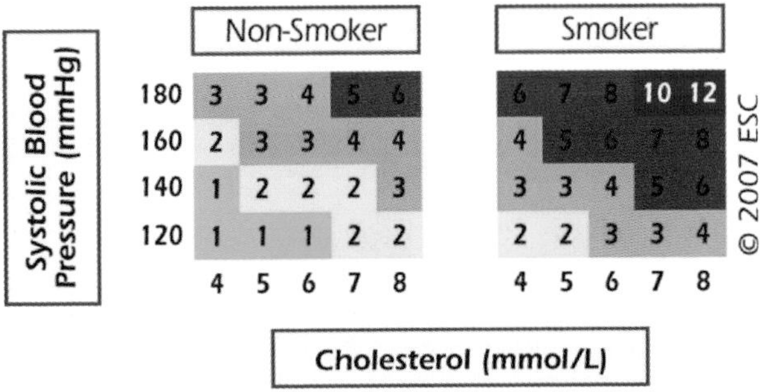

Plate 5 Relative risk chart. Reproduced from the original version of the European Guidelines on CVD Prevention. Executive Summary (European Heart Journal 2007;28:2375-2414) and Full text (European Journal) of Cardiovascular Prevention and Rehabilitation 2007;14 (suppl 2):S1-S113. Reproduction with permission of the European Society of Cardiology. © 2007 ESC. (see fig 1.1 p 11)

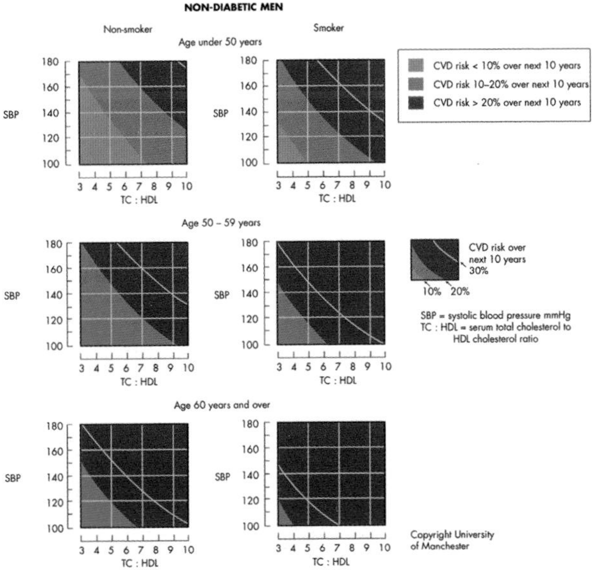

Plate 6 Joint British Societies' CVD risk prediction chart: non-diabetic men. (See fig 1.2 p 14)

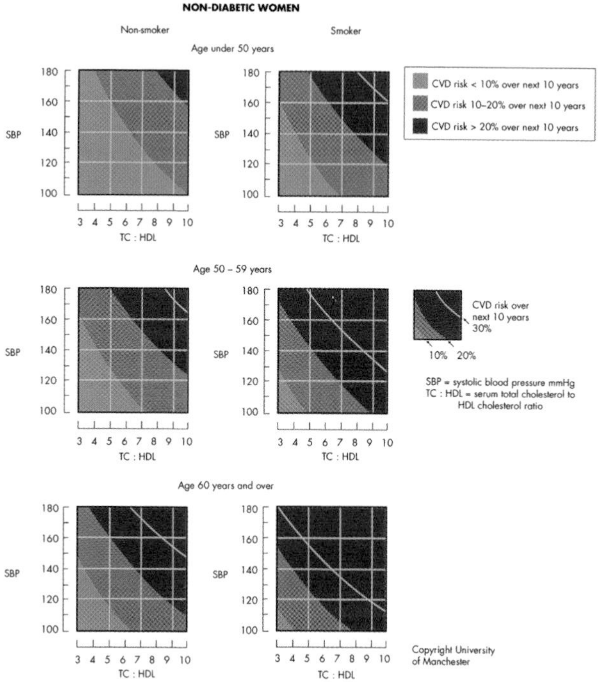

Plate 7 Joint British Societies' CVD risk prediction chart: non-diabetic women. (See fig 1.3 p 15)

How to assess risk

- Those with:
  - known CHD or other major atherosclerotic disease
  - type 2 diabetes or type 1 diabetes with microalbuminuria
  - very high levels of individual risk factors
  - familial hypercholesterolaemia or other inherited dyslipidaemias

  are already at INCREASED CVD RISK and need management of all risk factors.
- For all other people, the risk charts can be used to estimate total risk because many people have mildly raised levels of several risk factors that, in combination, can result in unexpectedly high levels of total CVD risk.

The charts are an aid to making clinical decisions about how intensively to intervene on lifestyle and whether to use antihypertensive, lipid-lowering, and antiplatelet medication, but should not replace clinical judgement.

Box 1.1 Advantages of using the risk charts

- Intuitive, easy to use tool.
- Takes account of the multifactorial nature of CVD.
- Estimates risk of all atherosclerotic CVD, not just CHD.
- Allows flexibility in management—if an ideal risk-factor level cannot be achieved, total risk can still be reduced by reducing other risk factors.
- Allows a more objective assessment of risk over time.
- Establishes a common language of risk for clinicians.
- Shows how risk increases over age.
- The relative risk chart helps to illustrate how a young person with a low absolute risk may be at a substantially higher and reducible relative risk.

JES4: SCORE risk estimation system

The SCORE system[3] estimates the 10-year risk of a first fatal atherosclerotic event (heart attack, stroke, aneurysm of the aorta, or other). Everyone with a 10-year risk of CVD death of 5% or more has an increased risk considered to be sufficiently high to justify intensive lifestyle interventions and, where appropriate, the use of drug therapies.

Box 1.2 How to use the SCORE charts to assess total CVD risk in asymptomatic persons

- Use the low-risk chart in Belgium*, France, Greece*, Italy, Luxemburg, Spain*, Switzerland, and Portugal; use the high-risk chart in other countries in Europe. *Updated, re-calculated charts are now available for Belgium, Germany, Greece, The Netherlands, Spain, Sweden, and Poland.
- Find the cell nearest to the person's age, cholesterol and BP values, bearing in mind that the risk will be higher as the person approaches the next age, cholesterol or BP category.
- Check the qualifiers.
- Establish the total 10-year risk for fatal CVD. Note that a low total cardiovascular risk in a young person may conceal a high relative risk; this may be explained to the person by using the relative risk chart. As the person ages, a high relative risk will translate into a high total risk. More intensive lifestyle advice will be needed in such persons.

Box 1.3 Risk estimation using SCORE: qualifiers

- The charts should be used in the light of the clinician's knowledge and judgement, especially with regard to local conditions.
- As with all risk estimation systems, risk will be overestimated in countries with a falling CVD mortality rate, and underestimated if it is rising.
- At any given age, risk appears lower for women than men. This is misleading since, ultimately, more women than men die from CVD. The risk for women is merely deferred by 10 years.
- Risk may be higher than indicated in the chart in:
  - sedentary or obese subjects, especially those with central obesity
  - subjects with a strong family history of premature CHD
  - the socially deprived
  - subjects with diabetes—the risk may be fivefold higher in women with diabetes and threefold higher in men with diabetes, compared to those without diabetes
  - subjects with low HDL cholesterol or high triglycerides
  - asymptomatic subjects with evidence of preclinical atherosclerosis; for example, a reduced ankle–brachial index or on imaging, such as carotid ultrasonography or computed tomography (CT) scanning.

The SCORE risk charts are shown in Plates 1–4 (see colour plate section).

Relative risk chart

The relative risk chart may be used to show younger people that, even if their absolute risk is low, it may still be many times higher than that of a person of a similar age with low risk factors. This may help to motivate decisions about avoidance of smoking, healthy eating, and exercise, as well as flagging those who may become candidates for medication (Fig. 1.1).
The HeartScore is the electronic and interactive version of the SCORE risk charts, aiming to provide physicians and patients with information on how total risk can be both estimated and reduced by lifestyle and therapeutic interventions. It is available at www.escardio.org/prevention.

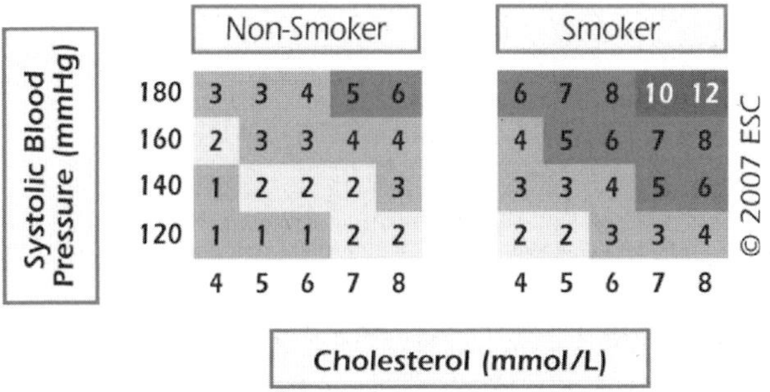

Fig. 1.1 Relative risk chart. Reproduced from the original version of the European Guidelines on CVD Prevention. Executive Summary (*European Heart Journal* 2007;28:2375-2414) and Full text (*European Journal of Cardiovascular Prevention and Rehabilitation* 2007;14 (suppl 2):S1-S113). Reproduced with permission of the European Society of Cardiology. © 2007 ESC. (See Plate 5)

JBS2: CVD risk prediction chart

The JBS2[4] CVD prediction chart estimates the total 10-year risk of developing CVD. A total CVD risk ≥ 20% over 10 years is considered sufficiently high to justify intensive lifestyle interventions and, where appropriate, the use of drug therapies.

Box 1.4 How to use the JBS2 CVD risk prediction charts in asymptomatic persons

- To estimate an individual's total 10-year risk of developing CVD, choose the table for his or her sex, lifetime smoking status, and age. Within this square, define the level of risk according to the point where the coordinates for systolic blood pressure and the ratio of total cholesterol to HDL cholesterol meet. If no HDL cholesterol result is available, then assume that this is 1.0 mmol/l.
- Smoking status should reflect lifetime exposure to tobacco use at the time of assessment. Those who have given up smoking within 5 years should be regarded as current smokers for the purposes of the charts.
- CVD risk should be estimated for person's current age group: <50, 50–59, or >60 years. For people under 40 years the CVD risk will be overestimated because the chart is based on risk at age 49 years. For people aged 70 and over the CVD risk will be underestimated because it is based on age 69 years.
- Check the qualifiers.

Box 1.5 Risk estimation using the JBS2 CVD risk prediction charts: qualifiers

- The charts should be used in the light of the clinician's knowledge and judgement.
- CVD risk is higher than indicated in the charts for:
  - family history of premature CVD or stroke (male first-degree relatives aged <55 years and female first-degree relatives aged <65 years), which increases the risk by a factor of approximately 1.4
  - South Asian origin: increases the risk by 1.5
  - serum triglycerides of 1.7 mmol/l or more: increases the risk by 1.3
  - impaired fasting glycaemia (in the range 6.1–6.9 mmol/l): increases the risk by 1.5
  - women with premature menopause.

The JBS2 risk prediction charts are shown in Figs 1.2 and 1.3

The Joint British Societies CVD risk assessor is the electronic and interactive version for estimating CVD risk. It is an aid to making clinical decisions about how intensively to intervene on lifestyle and whether to use cardioprotective drug therapies. It is available on www.access2information.org/health/cvra

3 Graham, I., Atar, D., Borch-Johnsen, K. *et al.* (2007). European guidelines on cardiovascular disease prevention in clinical practice: full text. Fourth Joint Task Force of the European Society of Cardiology and other Societies on Cardiovascular Disease Prevention in Clinical Practice. *European Journal of Cardiovascular Prevention and Rehabilitation*, **14**(Suppl 2), S1–S113.

4 British Cardiac Society, British Hypertension Society, Diabetes UK, HEART UK, Primary Care Cardiovascular Society, The Stroke Association. JBS2 (2005) Joint British Societies' guidelines on prevention of cardiovascular disease in clinical practice. *Heart*, **91**(Suppl V), V1–V5.

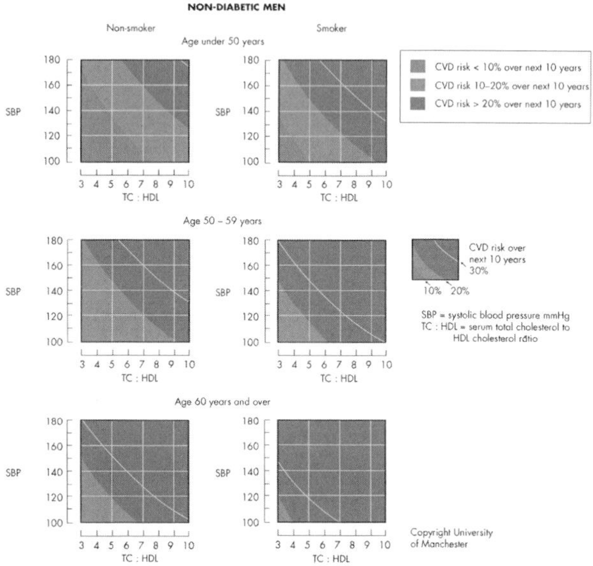

Fig. 1.2 Joint British Societies' CVD risk prediction chart: non-diabetic men. (See Plate 6)

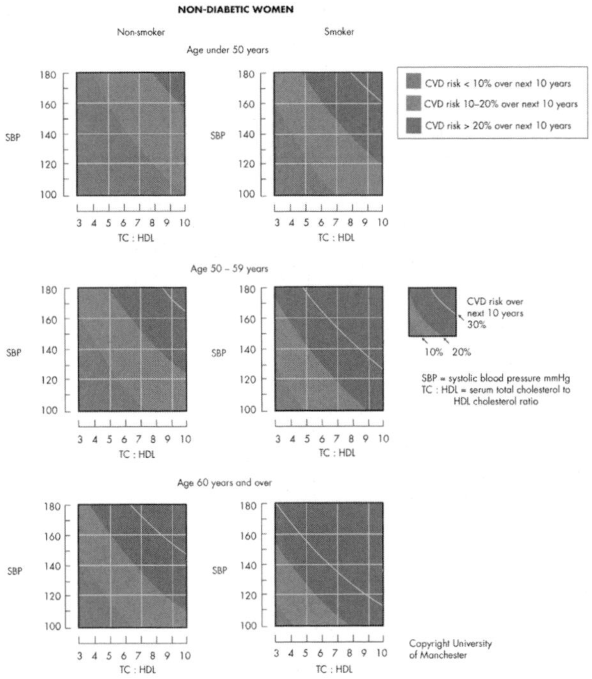

Fig. 1.3 Joint British Societies' CVD risk prediction chart: non-diabetic women. (See Plate 7)

Why families too?

- Some studies have confirmed that couples share the same lifestyle and risk factors.
- Whilst positive family history has been shown to be an independent risk factor for coronary heart disease, the relationship between family history and the incidence of disease in families is also a result of the aggregation of the major risk factors, for example raised blood pressure, raised cholesterol, diabetes, resulting from a shared lifestyle.
- Family aggregation of risk factors is partly determined by 'assortative mating', in other words, individuals are more likely to select mates who have the same characteristics as themselves ('like marries like'). Following this selection, couples go on to share lifestyle habits over a prolonged period which may contribute to reinforcing the continuing presence of risk factors in both.
- Partners (spouses) and first-degree relatives of patients with atherosclerotic disease are at higher risk of developing cardiovascular disease than the general population.
- People do not exist in isolation. They are part of a social network which includes their close family, friends, and carers.
- Family members living in the same household can support each other to make healthy lifestyle changes.

Table 1.2 Involvement of families in preventive cardiology programmes

Benefits	Considerations
• Positive social support from the family facilitates lifestyle changes, for example: the person responsible for buying and cooking food is actively involved in the programme and will therefore have a clear understanding of the principles of a cardioprotective diet • The family members benefit from the programme and reduce their cardiovascular disease risk • Families can discuss the programme together when they are at home and away from it, and remind each other of their goals, which may improve compliance with treatments and increase motivation • A truthful picture of lifestyle habits is more likely to emerge as a result of family members attending the programme • Lifestyle change is more likely to be sustained in the long term because of the continuing social support provided by family members	• The patient may not want their family members to be involved • People need their own space • Patients who live alone and cannot bring a family member with them may feel compromised

Key references

De Sutter, J., De Bacquer, D., Kotseva, K., *et al.* on behalf of the EUROASPIRE II Study Group. (2003). Screening family members of patients with premature coronary heart disease. *European Heart Journal*, **24**(3), 249–57.

Kolonel, L.N. and Lee, J. (1981). Husband–wife correspondence in smoking, drinking, and dietary habits. *American Journal of Clinical Nutrition*, **34**, 99–104.

Pyke, S., Wood, D.A., Kinmonth, A.L., and Thompson, S. (1997). Concordance of changes in coronary risk and risk factor levels in couples following lifestyle intervention in the British Family Heart Study. *Archives of Family Medicine*, **6**(4), 354–60.

Wood, D., Roberts, T., and Campbell, M. (1997). Women married to men with myocardial infarction are at increased risk of coronary heart disease. *Journal of Cardiovascular Risk*, **4**, 7–11.

Chapter 2

The nurse-led multidisciplinary team

The core team in a preventive cardiology programme

A team by definition is a group of people working toward a common goal. The overall goal of the preventive cardiology programme multidisciplinary team is to achieve and sustain key lifestyle changes, risk factor and therapeutic targets.

- The programme is co-ordinated by a specialist nurse with support from a dedicated cardiologist, general practitioner, dietitian and physiotherapist/ physical activity specialist (Fig. 2.1).
- The professionals working in the core team should have dedicated time for running the programme. The minimum recommendation is for one full-time nurse, a half-time dietitian, a half-time physiotherapist or physical activity specialist and 2 hours per week of dedicated physician time.
- With this level of staffing it should be possible to recruit 150 families in a year.
- Many other disciplines are also involved but are accessed as appropriate to individual needs.
- A strong sense of co-ordination, integration, and teamwork is needed in order to optimize outcomes in patients, their partners, and relatives.

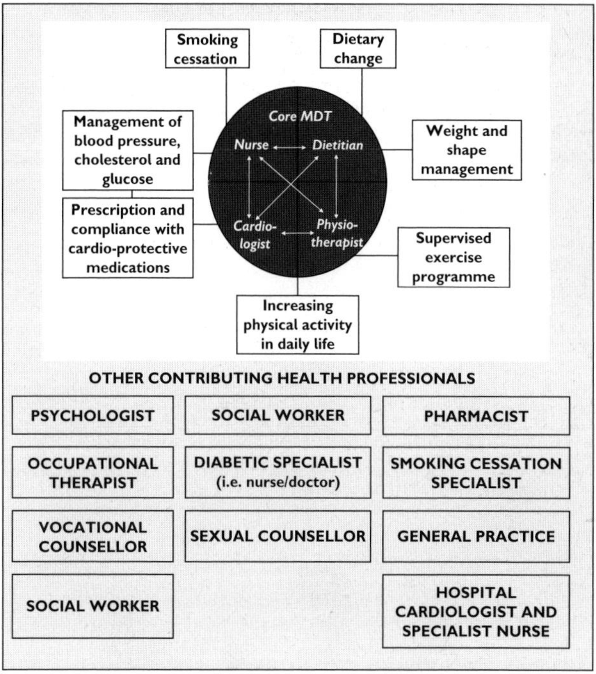

Fig. 2.1 The multidisciplinary team.

The evidence and justification for multidisciplinary working in cardiovascular disease prevention and rehabilitation

- Programmes that include a comprehensive multidisciplinary approach bringing together behavioural modification principles, exercise training, and optimal pharmacotherapy have been shown to be effective in achieving lifestyle, risk factor, and therapeutic targets in patients with coronary disease.[1,2,3]
- Targeting interventions at high-risk individuals and not at the general population is probably more effective.[4]
- The British Association for Cardiac Rehabilitation (BACR) Standards[5] endorse a dedicated core team consisting of cardiologists, nurses, dietitians, and physiotherapists.
- The ethos of including a multidisciplinary team is that this model of care offers a range of knowledge and skills.
    - With the complexity of service required there is a need for a range of disciplines, offering a wide scope of the knowledge and skills to address the breadth of physical, social, and psychological needs.
    - The core disciplines are best placed to facilitate a change in lifestyle in the three key areas of smoking, poor dietary habits, and physical inactivity. However, the service should also embrace the disciplines of health promotion, behavioural psychology, clinical psychology, pharmacy, and occupational therapy.

1 Taylor, R., Brown, A., Ebrahim, S, *et al.* (2004). Exercise based rehabilitation for patients with coronary heart disease: systematic review and meta-analysis of randomised controlled trials. *American Journal of Medicine*, **116**, 682–692.

2 Wood, D.A., Kotseva, K., Connolly, S. *et al.*, on behalf of EUROACTION Study Group. (2008). Nurse-coordinated multidisciplinary, family-based cardiovascular disease prevention programme (EUROACTION) for patients with coronary heart disease and asymptomatic individuals at high risk of cardiovascular disease: a paired, cluster-randomised controlled trial. *Lancet*, **371**, 1999–2012

3 Haskell, W.J., Alerman, E.L,. Fair, JM. (1994). Effects of intensive multiple risk factor reduction on coronary atherosclerosis and clinical cardiac events in men and women with coronary atherosclerosis and clinical cardiac events in men and women with coronary artery disease: the Stanford Coronary Risk Intervention Project (SCRIP). *Circulation*, **89**:975-990

4 Ebrahim, S., Beswick, A., Burke, M., and Davey Smith, G. (2006), *Multiple risk factor interventions for primary prevention of coronary heart disease*. Cochrane Database of Systematic Reviews.

5 BACR guidelines (June 2007). Available at http://www.bcs.com/documents/affiliates/bacr/BACR%20Standards%202007.pdf

The role of the nurse in a preventive cardiology programme

- The nurse is the programme co-ordinator and requires strong leadership, management (including budget) and communication skills. They should also possess a strategic vision for the programme.
- The nurse-coordinated approach to preventive care has been well documented.[2, 6–10]

A cardiac specialist nurse is an appropriate co-ordinator because he/she has training in the following skills:

- Implementing medical decisions about care.
- Monitoring signs and symptoms; for example, blood pressure.
- Safe administration of medicines (familiarity with medications, doses, potential interactions, and so on).
- An holistic and health-promoting approach rather than a disease-oriented approach to care.
- Medical, biological, social, and behavioural sciences, as well as health psychology.
- Management.
- Counselling and teaching.
- Coping with emotional problems (anger, fear, denial and dealing with death, dying, and loss).

However, like all professionals, these nurses are aware of the limits of their knowledge and recognize the need for referral to other disciplines when required. In the UK, the *Scope of Professional Practice* from the Nursing and Midwifery Council provides guidance on the necessity for professional updating and development through extra study and training, and also understanding the importance of recognizing limitations and knowing when it is appropriate to refer to other disciplines.

Box 2.1 The role of the nurse

- Coordinate and lead the programme whilst working as an integral part of the multidisciplinary team.
- Liaise with inpatient services (e.g. coronary care), outpatient services (e.g. cardiology clinics), primary care practices, and other necessary services to identify and recruit patients and families to the programme; proactive identification and recruitment to the programme of all eligible patients and their families.
- Provide cardiovascular nursing expertise.
- Provide individual nursing assessment of patients and families for cardiovascular risk factors at the start and end of the programme and for long-term follow up.
- Provide one-to-one support to patients and families as required.
- Coordinate the regular multidisciplinary review of all patients and families participating in the programme.
- Demonstrate specialist skills and behavioural strategies to facilitate smoking cessation.
- Monitor cardiovascular risk factors (blood pressure, lipids, and glucose) and liaise with the cardiologist/physician to review and appropriately titrate cardioprotective and other drug therapies for those recruited to the programme. Ideally, the nurse is an independent nurse prescriber.
- Co-ordinate a programme of health promotional workshops and provide specialist nursing and preventive cardiology input into specific workshops.
- Provide nursing support and advanced life support if required at the supervised exercise training sessions of the programme.
- Facilitate behaviour change for all components of the preventive cardiology programme in all patients/relatives/partners by active participation in health promotion.
- Ensure that resources are monitored and utilized effectively and appropriately.
- Ensure effective liaison with hospital cardiologist, where appropriate, and the general practitioner, to ensure continuity of preventive care in the long term.

6 Murchie, P. *et al.* (2003). RCT of secondary prevention clinics for coronary heart disease in primary care. *British Medical Journal*, **326**(7380), 84.

7 Murchie, P. *et al.* (2005). RCT of secondary prevention clinics for coronary heart disease in primary care. *British Medical Journal*, **330**(7493), 707.

8 Moher, M. *et al.* (2001). RCT to compare three methods of promoting secondary prevention of CHD in primary care. *British Medical Journal*, **322**(7298), 1338.

9 Cupples, M. et al. (1994). RCT Health Promotion in General Practice. British Medical Journal, **309**(6960), 993–996.

10 Cupples, M. et al. (1999). RCT Health Promotion in General Practice. British Medical Journal, **319**, 687–688.

The role of the dietitian and physiotherapist in a preventive cardiology programme

The dietitian

The dietitian is responsible for bringing specialist nutritional expertise to the preventive cardiology team. She or he is an integral member of the team and should have dedicated time to work on the programme. Dietitians use their expertise in conjunction with behavioural strategies to facilitate the adoption of a diet which promotes cardiovascular health, which helps to achieve and maintain a healthy blood pressure, lipid profile and good diabetic control, and which is consistent with achieving and maintaining a healthy weight and shape. The dietitian must take a holistic approach, focusing on all aspects that may affect dietary intake and adopt appropriate behaviour change strategies to promote change. The role of the dietitian is summarized in Box 2.2.

Box 2.2 The role of the dietitian

- Complete the dietetic assessment of all patients and families recruited to the programme at the start of the programme, at the end of the programme and in the long term.
- Contribute to the weekly multidisciplinary review of all patients and families participating in the programme.
- Provide one-to-one support to patients and families as required.
- Provide support and teaching to fellow team members so that skills can be transferred between professionals, where appropriate.
- Support the weekly health promotion workshop programme and deliver the dietary workshops.
- Attend the weekly programme meetings with patients and their families in order to follow up on lifestyle and risk factor management and support the supervised exercise session.
- To develop educational material for families to support dietary intervention.
- Refer to other specialists when necessary.
- To develop relationships with other service providers in the local area.
- To be aware of the local cultural, social, and deprivation mix.

The physiotherapist/physical activity specialist

The physiotherapist/physical activity specialist is responsible for bringing specialist expertise in physical activity and exercise to the preventive cardiology team. She or he is an integral member of the team and should have dedicated time to work on the programme. Physiotherapists/physical activity specialists use their expertise in conjunction with behavioural strategies to facilitate the adoption of an active lifestyle consistent with promoting cardiovascular health, achieving and maintaining a healthy blood pressure and lipid profile and good diabetic control, and with achieving and maintaining a healthy weight and shape.

The physiotherapist/physical activity specialist uses his or her knowledge and skills in assessing fitness and interpreting clinical exercise test results to develop safe and effective exercise and physical activity plans, sensitive to each individual's physical, psychosocial (cognitive and behavioural) capabilities, and needs. Physiotherapists/physical activity specialists also use their knowledge in pathophysiology in order to adapt and tailor exercises to the limitations and co-morbidities of patients and their family members. The physiotherapist/physical activity specialist takes a holistic approach, focusing on health promotion, rehabilitation, and performance enhancement to facilitate the achievement of individual goals, return to work, and normal activities. The role of the physiotherapist/physical activity specialist is summarized in Box 2.3.

Box 2.3 The role of the physiotherapist/physical activity specialist

- Complete the physical activity assessment of all patients and families recruited to the programme at the start of the programme, at the end of the programme and in the long term.
- Deliver the supervised exercise programme.
- Prescribe, monitor, and progress individualized home exercise and activity plans for all patients and families.
- Contribute to the weekly multidisciplinary review of all patients and families.
- Provide one-to-one support to patients and families as required.
- Provide support and teaching to fellow team members so that skills can be transferred between professionals, where appropriate.
- Support the weekly health promotion workshop programme and deliver the physical activity workshops.
- Attend the weekly programme meetings with patients and their families in order to follow up on lifestyle and risk-factor management and lead the supervised exercise session.
- Recruit community-based physical activity programmes suitable for this population group, thereby facilitating an active lifestyle in the long term.
- Provide long-term follow-up where indicated.
- Refer to other specialists where indicated (e.g. musculoskeletal physiotherapy).

Role of the cardiologist, general practitioner, and other physicians

Physician involvement in the programme

While the core multidisciplinary team is responsible for the delivery of the preventive cardiology programme, physician support, from a cardiologist or a physician with appropriate experience, is essential for the following areas.

- To review any new cardiac symptoms or change in functional status of the patient.
- To support the nurse in the medical management of blood pressure, lipids, and glucose, with attainment of recommended national targets.
- For the prescription and up-titration of appropriate cardioprotective therapies (if nurse prescriber not available).

Referral to other specialities, such as diabetology, should be considered if there is newly diagnosed diabetes or poor glycaemic control. Patients with significant health anxiety or symptoms of depression should have access to appropriate psychological support.

General practitioner

Engagement of the primary-care physician is important, as he or she is likely to be responsible for the identification and referral of individuals at high multifactorial risk. The longitudinal nature of their relationship with the patient should help promote uptake of the programme by the patient and their family, and also promote adherence. In addition, they are important for reinforcement of the programme's key messages.

The core team should also ensure regular communication and feedback to the patient's primary-care physician during the course of the programme. Communication with regards to achievements in lifestyle and medical risk-factor targets, with details of medication, is important so that the general practitioner can help the patient try to maintain these changes in the longer term.

For first-degree relatives of patients who present with premature coronary disease, the general practitioner has an essential role in screening for, assessing, and managing risk factors. The general practice team's collaboration is sought in achieving and maintaining cardiovascular lifestyle and other risk-factor targets in the long term.

Input of other disciplines to the preventive cardiology programme

While the core disciplines of nursing, dietetics, and physiotherapy are involved in the direct delivery of the preventive cardiology programme, they will need to refer to other disciplines. Some examples are listed below, but this list is not exhaustive. Hence, it is vital that the core team have good relations with, and spend time investigating, the wide range of services available within the hospital, primary-care setting, and the local community.

- ***Psychologist.*** The disciplines of clinical and health psychology can support the team in the following ways. Referral may sometimes be necessary for cases of moderate to severe anxiety and depression, particularly for coronary patients. It may also be possible for the psychologist to teach the team simple cognitive behavioural therapy techniques to help in the management of mild anxiety and depression. The advice of a health psychologist may be invaluable to the team, as this professional has an in-depth understanding of the psychosocial problems that accompany heart disease and is a specialist in the promotion of the adoption of healthy lifestyle behaviours. Psychologists may also be able to contribute to the group-based health promotion workshop programme where this service is available.
- ***Pharmacist.*** Ideally, a pharmacist should be available to provide information to patients and their families regarding their medications. This may result in improved compliance, increased efficacy, and optimization of drug regimes. Wherever possible, the pharmacist should deliver the group-based health promotion workshop session on cardioprotective medications for the programme. The programme nurse should establish useful links with either hospital-based or community pharmacists, and encourage patients and families to use their local pharmacist as a source of knowledge and support regarding their medications.
- ***Occupational therapist.*** Occupational therapists have the skills to facilitate groups on stress and anxiety management and teach relaxation techniques, as well as offering advice on activities of daily living, returning to work, leisure activities, and energy conservation. The health-promotion workshop programme can include sessions focused on stress-management techniques, which can be delivered by an occupational therapist where available.
- ***Addiction services.*** Heavily addicted smokers, for example, who have not responded to your smoking cessation service, may need more intensive support.
- ***Diabetic team.*** Patients or other family members with newly diagnosed or poorly controlled diabetes should be referred to the hospital or community diabetic team.
- ***Sexual counselor.*** Following the development of CVD all patients and their partners should be advised about resuming sexual activity. Referrals can also be made to an appropriate specialist for particular problems such as erectile dysfunction.
- ***Social worker.*** Cardiovascular disease and cardiovascular risk factors are linked to lower socio-economic status and thus to deprivation.

Patients from lower socio-economic groups may need an advocate in cases, for example, where they are forced into retirement, possibly unfairly, after a cardiac event. The social worker is well qualified to assist in this process and will play an important role in many individual cases.

- ***Vocational counselor.*** Some individuals may require special advice about returning to work after myocardial infarction and bypass surgery, for example.
- ***Other.*** Lay workers are involved where available, playing an important role in bridging the language and cultural divide sometimes found between health professionals and ethnically and culturally different patient populations. It can prove very effective in ethnic minorities, if a lay person speaking the language and familiar with cultural issues is involved.

Conclusion

The core multidisciplinary team ideally comprises a nurse co-ordinator, a dietitian, and physiotherapist/physical activity specialist who commit dedicated time to the programme, and have support from a cardiologist or other physician. This allows the programme to address three key lifestyle behaviours: abstinence from tobacco, healthy food choices, and being physically active; and also to facilitate management to target of cardiovascular risk factors. These core disciplines collaborate and work as a team, integrating an effective lifestyle management programme for patients and their families. However, the service also embraces other disciplines of health promotion—behavioural psychology, clinical psychology, pharmacy, and occupational therapy to name but a few. These other disciplines support the health promotion group based workshops and are accessed through referral should the comprehensive multidisciplinary assessment highlight the need for the input of their specialized skills. This highly professional multidisciplinary approach allows the development of an individualized and comprehensive programme for each patient and family attending the programme.

Chapter 3

Identification and recruitment

Priority groups for CVD prevention

- People with any form of established atherosclerotic CVD.
- Asymptomatic people without established CVD but with risk factor combinations putting them at high total risk of developing atherosclerotic CVD.
- People with diabetes mellitus (type 1 or 2).
- Markedly elevated single risk factors with target organ damage.
- Familial dyslipidaemia, such as familial hypercholesterolaemia or familial combined hyperlipidaemia.
- People with a family history of premature CVD (men <55 years, women <65 years).

The practicalities of recruitment

Patients with symptomatic atherosclerotic disease

Diagnostic categories

- Acute coronary syndrome (ST elevation myocardial infarction (STEMI), non-ST elevation myocardial infarction (NSTEMI); acute myocardial ischaemia).
- Exertional angina.
- Transient ischaemic attack (TIA).
- Peripheral arterial disease (PAD).

Where from?

- Hospital Coronary Care Unit (CCU) or other acute admission areas (e.g. cardiac catheterization, cardiology, and cardiac surgery units).
- Acute coronary syndrome nurse.
- Rapid access chest pain clinic.
- Hospital or community based TIA or vascular clinic.
- Other ambulatory hospital services.
- Community-based cardiology services.
- General practice.

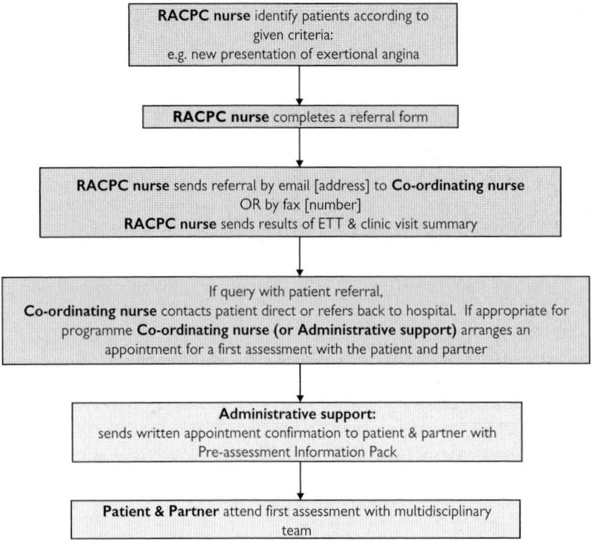

Fig. 3.1 Example of a referral pathway: from rapid access chest pain clinic (RACPC) to the preventive cardiology programme.

Box 3.1 An example of pre-screening criteria that may facilitate the identification of people at high CVD risk

- Men and women with no atherosclerotic disease with **one** or more of the pre-screening criteria specified below (men), and **two** or more of the pre-screening criteria specified below (women) should have their total CVD risk estimated.
  - Current tobacco smoker
  - Raised blood pressure (≥140/90 mmHg)
  - Raised blood lipids (total cholesterol ≥5 mmol/l)
- Patients ≥40 years who meet the pre-screening criteria defined above should have their cardiovascular risk estimated. If CVD risk is ≥20% (JBS2) or ≥5% (SCORE) over 10 years, they are eligible for the preventive cardiology programme.

People at high risk of developing cardiovascular disease

Diagnostic categories

- Asymptomatic people without established CVD but with risk-factor combinations putting them at high total risk of developing atherosclerotic CVD.
- People with diabetes mellitus (type 1 or 2).
- Markedly elevated single risk factors with target organ damage.
- Familial dyslipidaemia, such as familial hypercholesterolaemia or familial combined hyperlipidaemia.
- People with a family history of premature CVD (men <55 years, women <65 years).

Where from?

- General practice
- Polyclinics
- Specialist ambulatory clinics in hospital or community (e.g. diabetes, hypertension, lipid, obesity, etc.)

How to identify patients

- Use risk estimation tools to identify asymptomatic people without established atherosclerotic CVD but with multiple risk factors. Chapter 1 of this manual provides an explanation of how to calculate risk using the British (JBS2) and European (SCORE) risk estimation tools.
- Give general practices criteria that they can use to identify people who may be at sufficiently high risk to warrant entry to a preventive cardiology programme.

Partners and other members of the same household as the patient

- Invite all the partners and other family members living in the same household as the patient to join the preventive cardiology programme.

First-degree relatives of patients who present with premature atherosclerotic CVD

- Identify the first-degree relatives of recruited patients who present with premature coronary disease.

- Premature coronary disease is defined as developing before the age of 55 years in men and 65 years in women.
- First-degree relatives are the siblings and offspring of the patient with atherosclerotic CVD.

Box 3.2 Successful recruitment of patients and their families to the preventive cardiology programme will depend on the following

- Identifying specific sources of referral; for example, CCU, cardiology or acute medical ward, rapid access chest pain clinic, general practices, other vascular services (e.g. TIA clinic).
- Developing clear patient identification criteria and recruitment pathways from these sources to the programme.
- Identifying specific staff at the source referral sites who will liaise with the co-ordinating nurse on the preventive cardiology programme.
- Good communication between the co-ordinating nurse and the referral source.
- Clear division of responsibilities for those professionals who will play a part in the referral pathway.

IT IS IMPORTANT TO . . .

- Involve others who are delivering care to the same priority groups; for example, existing cardiac rehabilitation programmes or diabetes services.
- Join forces with these groups to ensure the provision of integrated care and no duplication of services.
- Monitor recruitment and talk with the source referral departments regularly to keep momentum going.

TIMELY RECRUITMENT

- Recruit patients and their families to the programme as soon as possible following their diagnosis, cardiac event, or being identified as being at high risk.

WHY?

- Capture the 'teachable moment', the beginning of the 'wake-up call', i.e. the time when the patient and family are most likely to be motivated to change behaviour and take action to reduce their risk.

Chapter 4

Comprehensive multidisciplinary family-based cardiovascular assessment

Principles of the multidisciplinary assessment of high-risk families

The preventive cardiology programme for each patient and family member should be based on a multifactorial assessment of:

- lifestyle (smoking, diet, physical activity)
- body weight and fat distribution
- blood pressure, blood lipids, blood glucose
- psychosocial status.

- Encourage couples (high-risk patient and their partner) to attend the assessment together.
- Each patient and family member invited to the assessment should be assessed by the nurse, the dietitian and the physiotherapist/physical activity specialist on the programme multidisciplinary team.

Assessment Timing

BASELINE

⇩

END OF PROGRAMME

⇩

ONE YEAR

Fig. 4.1 Timing of the assessment.

- An assessment at the start of the programme allows identification of problems and goals to be set.
- Once the intensive lifestyle and risk-factor programme is completed, a second assessment evaluates the immediate impact of the programme.
- A final assessment between 6 months and 1 year later will evaluate the longer-term impact of the programme.

Logistics of the assessment

- This detailed assessment can take up to 3 hours to complete for a couple.
- Maximizing the time dedicated by each professional is best achieved by organizing the assessment in the way shown in Fig. 4.2.
- In this way three couples can be assessed, for example, during a 3–4 hour period.

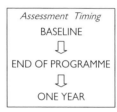

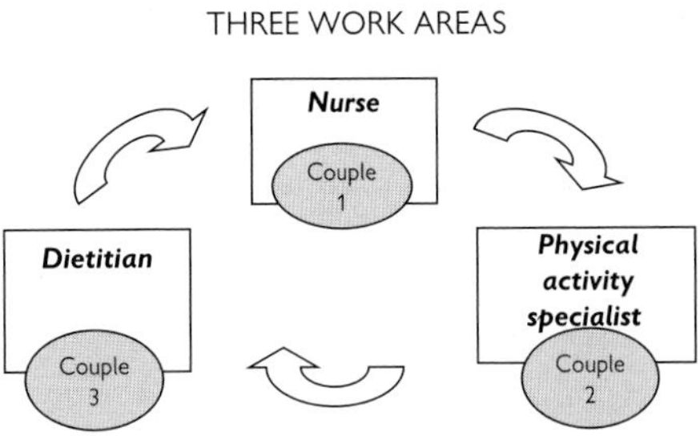

Fig. 4.2 The logistics of the multidisciplinary family assessment.

- Once the initial assessment is complete, the next stage is to agree goals for lifestyle change and other cardiovascular risk factors with the patient and their partner according to the problems you have identified together during the assessment, and according to their expectations and their priorities. Goal setting is described in more detail in Chapter 5.

Box 4.1 Outcome measures

- Proportions of patients achieving national lifestyle, risk factor and therapeutic targets for cardiovascular disease prevention:
  - smoking
  - diet/nutrition
  - physical activity
  - overweight/obesity
  - blood pressure
  - blood lipids and glucose
  - diabetes
  - prophylactic drug therapies
  - compliance with therapies
- Psychosocial
  - health-related quality of life
  - risk perception
  - illness perception
  - functional limitation
- Return to work
- Service use

Assessment of lifestyle

The next three sections of this chapter are devoted to describing methodologies for assessing lifestyle habits (smoking, diet, and physical activity). A variety of methodologies are described and evaluated. The final choice of tools used to assess these aspects of lifestyle should meet the following criteria:

- Answer the question
- Be reproducible
- Be valid for the particular population
- Be easy to use in the clinical setting.

Table 4.1 Assessing lifestyle

Lifestyle habit	Assessment tool
Smoking	Reported smoking status
	Objective validation of reported smoking status
	Stage of change
	Nicotine dependence
Diet	Food habits
	Dietary recall and analysis
	Anthropometric measures (weight, height, waist)
Physical activity	Physical activity in daily life
	Objective measure of reported physical activity
	Functional capacity
	Functional limitations

Considerations

- Standardized measurement of diet and physical activity is particularly problematic due to their complex and multidimensional natures.
- Measurement is often limited by the subjective nature of patient recall methodology.
- Objective measures are available for some aspects of lifestyle but these are often expensive and labour intensive.
- It is advisable to use a combination of subjective and objective measures and a multitude of tools which will facilitate a full investigation of each aspect of lifestyle.

Assessment of smoking

Designing an effective smoking cessation intervention depends on a comprehensive assessment of smoking status, readiness to quit, motivation, smoking in the family, a history of past quit attempts, psychological co-morbidities, and dependence on nicotine.

- ***Smoking status***: Ask all patients and their partners about smoking. Do they smoke now? Did they ever smoke? How many years have they smoked in their lives?
- ***Validating smoking status***: Use a biochemical marker to validate self-report as it increases its accuracy. Breath carbon monoxide is a practical and economical tool to use in a clinical setting. Table 4.2 shows the advantages and disadvantages of different approaches to assess smoking status.

Table 4.2 Assessing smoking status

Method	Advantages	Disadvantages
Self-report	Simple Time-efficient Inexpensive Non-invasive	Depends on honesty Does not take into account unintentional imprecision re. smoking habits
Expired carbon monoxide	Practical Not very costly Immediate results May help motivate	Short half-life Levels may increase in inflammatory lung conditions
Cotinine (urinary, saliva, blood)	Longer sensitivity time Correlates better with degree of smoking More accurate	Costly More invasive May be affected by concurrent nicotine replacement therapy (NRT) use

Box 4.2 Measuring breath carbon monoxide

For an accurate and reliable reading of the level of carbon monoxide in the breath, ensure the following:

- The manufacturer's instructions are read carefully.
- The correct procedure is explained to the individual.
- One reading is usually sufficient unless the first measurement is not completed in a satisfactory manner.
- The individual should understand that they should take in a breath and hold it during the countdown (15 seconds).

When the countdown has finished, the individual should be asked to seal their lips around the mouthpiece and to breathe out steadily and gently through it, emptying the lungs as much as possible.

- ***Motivation***: A more detailed explanation of assessing readiness and motivation to quit is provided in Chapter 5 of this manual. Table 4.3 (below) shows a way to assess 'stage of change' in a smoker.
- ***Family smoking status***: Do any of the other members of the family living at home with the patient and partner smoke? It is important to establish what positive social support is available within the family and in the immediate social environment for quit attempts to be successful.
- ***Past quit attempts***: Has the patient or partner tried to quit in the past? Ask about the adequacy of previous therapies and the perceived causes of lapses.
- ***Psychiatric co-morbidities***: Quitting smoking can precipitate depression in susceptible individuals. Ask whether there is a history of depression or other psychiatric morbidity.

Table 4.3 Assessing stage of change for smoking behaviour

Question	Answer	Stage
Have you ever smoked?	No	Non-smoker
	Quit	Go to last question
	Now	Go to next question
Do you intend to quit in 6 months and have you tried to quit for at least 24 hours in the last year?	No	Pre-contemplation
	Yes	Go to next question
If YES, are you ready to quit within 1 month?	Yes	Preparation
	No	Contemplation
If you quit, did you quit within the last 6 months?	Yes	Action
	No	Maintenance

Is the patient ready to stop smoking?	**Stage of change**	
	Non smoker	
	Pre-contemplation Contemplation	Ask about smoking status on ongoing basis
	Preparation Action	Arrange follow-up
	Maintenance	

- ***Dependence on nicotine***: How physically dependent is the patient/partner on nicotine? The Fagerström Test for Nicotine Dependence (FTND)[1] provides a validated tool to measure physical dependence (Table 4.4).

Table 4.4 Assessing nicotine dependence with the FTND

Is the patient nicotine dependent?	FTND score: /10	
	1–4 Low dependence	
	5–6 Moderate	
	>7 High	
Fagerstrom Test for Nicotine Dependence		
1. How soon after you wake up do you smoke your first cigarette?	Within 5 minutes	3
	6–30 minutes	2
	31–60 minutes	1
	After 60 minutes	0
2. Do you find it difficult to refrain from smoking in places where it is forbidden?	Yes	1
	No	0
3. Which cigarette would you hate to give up most?	The first one in the morning	1
	All others	0
4. How many cigarettes per day do you smoke?	10 or less	0
	11–20	1
	21–30	2
	31 or more	3
5. Do you smoke more frequently during the first hours after waking than during the rest of the day?	Yes	1
	No	0
6. Do you smoke if you are so ill that you are in bed most of the day?	Yes	1
	No	0
	Total	

1 Heatherton, T. *et al.* (1991). The Fagerström Test for Nicotine Dependence: a revision of the Fagerström Tolerance Questionnaire. *British Journal of Addiction*, **86**, 1119–27.

Assessment of diet and weight

Background to dietary assessments[2]

Dietary intake has many different influences. These influences will vary between individuals. Developing an understanding of these influences is essential to complete a detailed and accurate assessment.

Therefore, prior to or during the assessment the following factors should be addressed and taken into consideration to ensure that the appropriate assessment is completed.

Identification of assessment purpose

- Assess overall dietary balance and pattern.
- Identify level of consumption of specific foods, or groups of foods.
- Obtain a quantitative estimate of energy and/or nutrient intake.
- Identify nutritional deficiencies or surpluses.
- Identify food-related symptoms.
- Assess risk of malnutrition or overeating/drinking.
- Monitor compliance with dietary advice.

Oral intake is influenced by many different factors. When trying to establish a typical dietary intake of a person/family it is essential to consider possible influences that may affect food choice and to establish daily variation in terms of both frequency and quantity.

Factors affecting food choices

- Cultural background
- Religious or ethical beliefs
- Psychological (rewarding, punishing, comfort eating)
- Appetite level
- Taste preferences
- Financial issues
- Lifestyle/work hours and commitments (e.g. shift work, business travel/entertaining, type of work and hence availability of access to food/beverages)
- Difference between week days and weekends
- Social conventions/how food eaten (e.g. in front of TV; sat as family at a table; 'on the move')
- Meals taken outside of the home
- Family/peer group pressures
- Advertising
- Knowledge/beliefs about food and diet
- Previous advice given
- Previous diet attempts
- Weight history (fluctuations, stable, gradual gain or loss, yo-yo dieting)
- Available facilities

2 Thomas, B., Bishop, Y. (2007). Manual of dietetic practice. 4th ed. Blackwell.

Readiness to change

Changing dietary habits of a lifetime can be very difficult. All subjects should be assessed for their readiness and motivation to change. To be beneficial, dietary changes needs to be long term. Therefore all suggested changes should be realistic and achievable. For more information go to Chapter 5, Changing lifestyles.

Household influences

The dynamics of any household has a strong influence on the dietary habits of the people living within that house. Identification and collaboration with the person who is in charge of the food purchasing and food preparation is essential to improve outcome and long-term dietary change.

Habitual dietary assessment methods

Dietary habits are complex and very variable, leading to challenges in their measurement. Therefore the tools used need to be selected carefully. Not only is it essential to establish what is consumed, it is also important to gain an insight into the processes and feelings the family go through for food and drink selection, preparation, and consumption.

People are often sensitive about what they eat and drink. This can lead to reluctance and underestimation of what they perceive as 'bad' foods and overestimation of 'good' foods. To reduce this possible error it is important to ask open, indirect, or non-leading questions.

Closed question:	Do you have milk in coffee?
Open question:	How do you have your coffee?
Direct question:	How much butter do you use?
Indirect question:	How long does a pack of butter last you?
Leading question:	What do you have for breakfast?
Non-leading:	What would be the first thing you would eat or drink in the morning?

Obtaining dietary information with these methods of questioning in mind is essential. The quality of dietary modification advice relies completely on the quality and accuracy of the data collected in the assessment.

Possible methods of assessment of dietary intake: recall methods[3]

Food frequency questionnaire

Collection of data on the frequency a food or drink item is consumed and the amount eaten on each sitting. This is either interview led or completed by the participant.

24-hour recall

Interview-led recall collects information about the previous day's intake. Foods and drinks are described and portions estimated. Multiple days improve precision.

Diet history

Interview led, obtaining detailed information about usual foods and drinks consumed. Portion sizes, food preparation methods, and food frequency information are also collected.

Possible methods of assessment of dietary intake: record methods

Diet records/diaries

The participant records all that is eaten and drunk during a given period, most commonly 3 or 7 days. The portions are described either in household measures, weighed, in average portions, from photographs, or in pack sizes.

Checklist record

This is a list of food. Each time a participant eats a food he or she ticks it off the list and records the portion size consumed.

For advantages and disadvantages of each method see Appendix at the end of this section.

Portion size estimation

- It is essential to quantify the amount of food eaten.
- Portions of food are often difficult to quantify.
- Weighing each food item is the most accurate way although it is very labour intensive.
- Participant perception of what equals an average portion may vary.
- Underestimation of portion size is common, especially of those foods that are perceived to be bad.
- The use of photographs showing a variety of portions sizes can improve estimation.

Validation of assessment methods[3]

All types of dietary assessments on free-living subjects rely to varying extents on the ability of the subject to record or recall their intake. This provides a source of error, either through under- or overreporting or falsifications. Research has shown, for example, that those who are obese, female, or trying to lose weight will underreport their intake.

The best way to validate intake is by using biomarkers. Table 4.5 shows possible different biomarkers for different nutrients. These are often expensive, invasive, time consuming, and depend on the precision of the assays, so are rarely completed in clinical practice.

Table 4.5 Examples of biomarkers for reported nutrient validation

Nutrient	Possible biomarker
Energy intake	Doubly labelled water
Protein	24-hour nitrogen excretion in urine
n-3 fatty acids	Levels in adipose tissue or blood
Sodium and potassium	24-hour sodium and potassium excretion in urine
Antioxidants	Levels in plasma

3 Margetts, B., Nelson, M. (1997). Design concepts in nutritional epidemiology. 2nd ed. Oxford Medical Publications.

24-hour recall

In clinical practice, 24-hour dietary recall and diet history are the most frequently used tools. Below is a standardized method of completing a 24-hour recall.

Triple pass method[4]

Aim: to provide a complete record of all food and drink on the previous day between midnight and midnight.

The time element is important, as there may be people on shift work or with unusual time schedules whose dietary patterns are not typical.

The 24-hour recall is collected in three phases:[4]

1. A quick list of foods eaten or drunk

- Ask subjects to report everything that they had to eat or drink on the previous day between midnight and midnight.
- Do not interrupt.
- At the end of the recall, invite subjects to add any additional items not initially recalled.

2. Collection of detailed information concerning the items in the quick list

- For each item of food, you should ask the subjects to provide additional detail.
- Use open questioning.
- Ask subject to describe and quantify food in a consistent way:
  - type (salmon, lamb, cabbage, rice, potatoes)
  - state of food (canned, frozen, fresh)
  - cut of food (fillet, whole, slice, small pieces)
  - the cooking method (fried, roasted, boiled, steamed)
  - the amount eaten.
- Foods that are likely to be eaten in combination with other items should be prompted for
  - e.g. milk in coffee
  - sandwiches (fillings and bread)
  - pasta and salad.
- The quantity consumed should be based on household measures, food photographs, or named products.

3. A recall review

- Review all the food eaten and drunk in chronological order.
- Prompt for any additional eating occasions or foods possibly consumed and clarify any ambiguities regarding type of food eaten or portion size.
- ***Forgotten foods:*** ensure you ask specific questions on the following:
  - soft drinks
  - alcoholic drinks
  - sweets/chocolate/confectionery
  - crisps/nuts/other snacks
  - dressings/sauces
  - salt/pepper
  - dietary supplements.

A similar method can also be applied to a diet history methodology. Instead of asking about the past 24 hours the subject is asked what they normally would eat.

Energy requirements

Required information and formula

A person's estimated energy requirements to maintain body weight can be calculated using Schofield's formula (Box 4.3). For this calculation the following information is required:

- Weight (kg)
- Gender
- Age
- Activity level of the individual.

The figures in this formula are derived from the analysis of energy requirements commissioned by FAO/WHO/UNU (1985).[5]

The level of activity corresponds to the activity that the individual does **in addition** to the normal daily exertion involved in getting up, washing, going to work, attending meals, etc.

Light activity:	2 hours/day active on feet
Moderate activity:	6 hours/day active on feet
Heavy activity:	Reserved for a very heavy labouring and serious athletes in training

It is assumed that at least light activity will be encouraged for everybody. If this amount of additional exertion is not possible for medical or other reasons, then the energy requirement should be reduced by 15%.

4 Slimani, N., Deharveng, G., Charrondiere, R.U. *et al.* (1999). Structure of the standardized computerized 24-h diet recall interview used as reference method in the 22 centers participating in the EPIC project. European Prospective Investigation into Cancer and Nutrition. *Computer Methods and Programs in Biomedicine*, **58**(3), 251–66.

5 Schofield, W.N. (1985). Predicting basal metabolic rate, new standards and review of previous work. *Human Nutrition Clinical Nutrition*, **39**(Suppl 1), 5–41.

Box 4.3 Schofield's formula[6]

Men:
18–30 years: BMR[a] = 0.0630 × weight + 2.8957
31–60 years: BMR = 0.0484 × weight + 3.6534
60+ years: BMR = 0.0491 × weight + 2.4587

Women:
18–30 years: BMR = 0.0621 × weight + 2.0357
31–60 years: BMR = 0.0342 × weight + 3.5377
60+ years: BMR = 0.0377 × weight + 2.7545

Physical activity levels:

Inactive men and women	= BMR × 1.55	Activity Factor (AF)
Moderately active women	= BMR × 1.64	
Moderately active men	= BMR × 1.79	
Highly active women	= BMR × 1.82	
Highly active men	= BMR × 2.10	

[a] BMR, basal metabolic rate.

To convert to kcal (1 kcal = 4.2 kJ):

$$\frac{\text{BMR} \times \text{AF}}{4.2} \times 1000$$

Energy prescription for those with a weight loss target

For individuals who are trying to lose weight, 500 kcal should be subtracted from this figure to establish their target daily calorie intake.

6 Schofield, W.N., Schofield, C. and James, W.F.T. (1985). Basal metabolic rate. *Human Nutrition Clinical Nutrition*, **39C**(Suppl 1), 1–96.

Anthropometric measures

Anthropometric measurements provide predictions of body composition. This includes body mass, fat stores, and body water. A number of different measures are available for use. The accuracy, ease of use, time to complete, and cost of each measurement varies.

Normal parameters have been set for many of the different measures. (see Box 4.4). These norms are different for Asians (see Box 4.5).

Waist circumference (WC) and waist hip ratio (WHR)

WC and WHR are both measures of abdominal obesity and are the best anthropometric predictors of cardiovascular risk. A 1 cm increase in WC is associated with a 2% increase in risk of future CVD and a 0.01 increase in WHR is associated with a 5% increase in risk.

How to measure:

- Sit in front of the individual.
- Ensure the individual is standing straight with both feet together (supporting themselves on a piece of furniture if they cannot balance) looking straight ahead.
- Measure next to the skin or over one piece of light clothing.

To measure waist

- Measure midway between the lower rib margin and the iliac crest. (approx. 2.5 cm above the naval in many people).
- Mark the level of the lowest rib margin.
- Palpate the iliac crest in the mid-axillary line and mark it.
- Pass the tape horizontally around the subject's circumference mid way between the lowest rib margin and the iliac crest.
- The tape should be taut but not tight. Ensure that the individual is relaxed and breathing normally. Take measurement on expiration.

To measure hips

- Measure at the widest point around the hips and buttocks.

To calculate WHR

- Waist in inches/cm is divided by the hip measurement in inches/cm.

Height

- Measure without shoes, with the heels together and with the so-called Frankfurt plane of the head in a horizontal position.
- Ask the subject to breathe in deeply and reach up to a maximum height with the legs stretched and the feet flat on the ground. The height should be taken while the individual is looking straight ahead.
- Some weight scales have the height measure attached.

Weight

- Measure the subject while he or she is wearing light clothes. Ensure the removal of keys, phones, wallets, etc. from the subject's pockets.
- Both feet should be placed firmly on the centre of the scales.
- The scales should be calibrated yearly.

Body mass index (BMI)

This is an index of 'weight for height'. It is commonly used to classify underweight, overweight, and obesity in adults (Box 4.4). This World Health Organization (WHO) classification is based primarily on the association between BMI and mortality.

$$BMI = weight (kg)/ (height (m))^2$$

(Fig. 4.3 shows a graphical example).

The use of calculated BMI should be used with caution in the following subjects:

- Distorted fluid balance
- High proportion of muscle mass
- Problematic height measurement (spine curvation, loss of height in elderly)
- Enforced immobility.

Skin fold estimation method

This measures the relationship between subcutaneous fat and total body fat to estimate adiposity. It is not possible to measure visceral adipose tissue. Although it does not give an accurate reading of real body fat percentage, it is reliable at measuring a change of body composition over time.

Height (m)

Weight (kg)	1.43	1.46	1.5	1.53	1.56	1.59	1.62	1.65	1.68	1.71	1.74	1.77	1.8	1.83	1.86	1.89	1.92	1.95	1.96	Weight (St lbs)
146	71	68	65	62	60	58	56	54	52	50	48	47	45	44	42	41	40	38	37	23.0
143	70	67	64	61	59	57	54	53	51	49	47	46	44	43	41	40	39	38	36	22.5
139	68	65	62	59	57	55	53	51	49	48	46	44	43	42	40	39	38	37	35	21.9
136	67	64	60	58	56	54	52	50	48	47	45	43	42	41	39	38	37	36	35	21.4
133	65	62	59	57	55	53	51	49	47	45	44	42	41	40	38	37	36	35	34	20.9
130	64	61	58	56	53	51	50	48	46	44	43	41	40	39	38	36	35	34	33	20.5
127	62	60	56	54	52	50	48	47	45	43	42	41	39	38	37	36	34	33	32	20.0
124	61	58	55	53	51	49	47	46	44	42	41	40	38	37	36	35	34	33	32	19.5
120	59	56	53	51	49	47	46	44	43	41	40	38	37	36	35	34	33	32	31	18.9
117	57	55	52	50	48	46	45	43	41	40	39	37	36	35	34	33	32	31	30	18.4
114	56	53	51	49	47	45	43	42	40	39	38	36	35	34	33	32	31	30	29	18.0
111	54	52	49	47	46	44	42	41	39	38	37	35	34	33	32	31	30	29	28	17.5
108	53	51	48	46	44	43	41	40	38	37	36	34	33	32	31	30	29	28	28	17.0
105	51	49	47	45	43	42	40	39	37	36	35	34	32	31	30	29	28	28	27	16.5
101	49	47	45	43	42	40	38	37	36	35	33	32	31	30	29	28	27	27	26	15.9
98	48	46	44	42	40	39	37	36	35	34	32	31	30	29	28	27	27	26	25	15.4
95	46	45	42	41	39	38	36	35	34	32	31	30	29	28	27	27	26	25	24	15.0
92	45	43	41	39	38	36	35	34	33	31	30	29	28	27	27	26	25	24	23	14.5
89	44	42	40	38	37	35	34	33	32	30	29	28	27	27	26	25	24	23	23	14.0
86	42	40	38	37	35	34	33	32	30	29	28	27	27	26	25	24	23	23	22	13.5
83	41	39	37	35	34	33	32	30	29	28	27	26	26	25	24	23	23	22	21	13.1
82	40	38	36	35	34	32	31	30	29	28	27	26	25	24	24	23	22	22	21	12.9
79	39	37	35	34	32	31	30	29	28	27	26	25	24	24	23	22	21	21	20	12.4
76	37	36	34	32	31	30	29	28	27	26	25	24	23	23	22	21	21	20	19	12.0
73	36	34	32	31	30	29	28	27	26	25	24	23	23	22	21	20	20	19	19	11.5
70	34	33	31	30	29	28	27	26	25	24	23	22	22	21	20	20	19	18	18	11.0
66	32	31	29	28	27	26	25	24	23	23	22	21	20	20	19	18	18	17	17	10.4
63	31	30	28	27	26	25	24	23	22	22	21	20	19	19	18	18	17	17	16	9.9
60	29	28	27	26	25	24	23	22	21	21	20	19	19	18	17	17	16	16	15	9.5
57	28	27	25	24	23	23	22	21	20	19	19	18	18	17	16	16	15	15	15	9.0
54	26	25	24	23	22	21	21	20	19	18	18	17	17	16	16	15	15	14	14	8.5
51	25	24	23	22	21	20	19	19	18	17	17	16	16	15	15	14	14	13	13	8.0
48	23	23	21	21	20	19	18	18	17	16	16	15	15	14	14	13	13	13	12	7.6
45	22	21	20	19	18	18	17	17	16	15	15	14	14	13	13	13	12	12	11	7.1
41	20	19	18	18	17	16	16	15	15	14	14	13	13	12	12	11	11	11	10	6.5
40	20	19	18	17	16	16	15	15	14	14	13	13	12	12	12	11	11	11	10	6.3
Height (Ft In)	4.69	4.79	4.92	5.02	5.12	5.22	5.32	5.41	5.51	5.61	5.71	5.81	5.91	6.00	6.10	6.20	6.30	6.40	6.50	

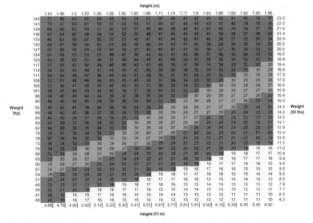

Fig. 4.3 BMI chart. Take a straight line across from your height (without shoes) and a line up from your weight. Put a mark where the two lines meet.

How to measure

- Take a pinch of skin at the triceps, biceps, subscapular, or iliac crest and measure with calipers. Take an average of several readings.
- Accuracy depends on a person's unique body fat distribution.

Possible error

- Movement of fat (as subject moves from sitting to standing).
- Inaccessibility of measurement site or subject too fat to measure.
- Fat distribution differs between individuals and can change differently.
- Sensitivity—large changes in weight are required to get changes in measurements.

Bioelectrical impedance analysis (BIA)

BIA is based on the principle that lean tissue is highly conductive to electrical current where as fat is more resistant. Measurement of the changes in voltages when a current is passed through electrodes results in a measurement of total body water. Total body water can be used to estimate fat-free body mass and, by difference with body weight, body fat.

Disadvantages

It depends on the subject's hydration levels and does not allow for differences in body geometry.

Recent technological improvements have made BIA a more reliable and therefore more acceptable way of measuring body composition. Nevertheless it is not a 'gold standard' or reference method.

Box 4.4 Parameters for anthropometric measures

Classification of adults according to BMI[a]

Classification	BMI	Risk of co-morbidities
Underweight	<18.50	Low (but risk of other clinical problems increased)
Normal range	18.50–24.99	Average
Overweight	≥25.00	
Preobese	25.00–29.99	Increased
Obese class I	30.00–34.99	Moderate
Obese class II	35.00–39.99	Severe
Obese class III	≥40.00	Very severe

Box 4.4 Parameters for anthropometric measures (*Continued*)

Sex-specific waist circumference and risk of metabolic complications associated with obesity in Caucasians[a]

Risk of metabolic complications	Waist circumference (cm) Men	Women
Increased	≥94	≥80
Substantially increased	≥102	≥88
Classification for waist hip ratio (WHR)		
Ideal WHR	<1.0	<0.85
Percentage body fat		
Acceptable percentage body fat	18–25%	25–31%

[a]WHO (2004). *Obesity: preventing and managing the global epidemic.* Report of a WHO Consultation. Geneva, World Health Organization. http://whqlibdoc.who.int/trs/WHO_TRS_894_(part1).pdf

Box 4.5 Co-morbidities risk associated with different levels of BMI and suggested waist circumference in adult Asians

Classification	BMI (kg/m^2)	Risk of co-morbidities	Waist circumference
		< 90 cm (men) < 80 cm (women)	≥ 90 cm (men) ≥ 80 cm (women)
Underweight	< 18.5	Low (but increased risk of other clinical problems)	Average
Normal range	18.5 - 22.9	Average	Increased
Overweight :	≥ 23		
At risk	23 - 24.9	Increased	Moderate
Obese I	25 - 29.9	Moderate	Severe
Obese II	≥ 30	Severe	Very severe

Inoue, S., Zimmet, P. et al. Feb 2000. *The asia-pacific perspective. Redefining obesity and its treatment.* http://www.diabetes.com.au/pdf/obesity_report.pdf

Appendix Advantages and disadvantages of different dietary assessment tools

Type of tool	Advantages	Disadvantages
Diet history	Obtains detailed information on a usual diet (meal pattern and food choice) Quick and simple Reduced effort required by subject as interview led Subject does not require literacy skills Does not affect food choice Possible to be completed over telephone Can cover weekdays, weekends, eating out and work influences	Interviewer requires training, skill dependent Under- or overestimation or fabrication of intake Relies on subject's ability to recall accurately Prone to interviewer bias Hard to standardize methodology
24-hour recall	Low in cost and quick to complete Assesses meal pattern and food choice Interview led More than one day improves precision Standardized methodology available Subject does not require literacy skills Does not affect food choice Detects dietary inadequacies/excesses and poor habits Possible to be completed over telephone	Only provides one day's information May not be representative of dietary pattern Dependent on interviewer's skills Relies on subject's ability to recall accurately

Food frequency questionnaire	Low in cost Easy to complete (self or interview administered) Uniformity of administration Analysis can be easy due ability of computer reading Good for large population studies (individuals categorized into quartiles of intake) Can examine food patterns or specific food groups over longer periods of time	Requires large amount of work for development and validation Can be large amounts of imprecision (over- and underestimation) Hard to identify which foods to include Questionnaire can take a very long time to complete Subject requires literacy skills Relies on subject's ability to recall accurately
Weighed diet record	If kept well, can be accurate Can achieve information for a number of days Weighing improves portion estimation Can also be used as a tool for treatment (highlights triggers to eating, dietary patterns,and quantity eaten) Can measure mean and standard deviation of nutrient intake	High workload for subject (weighing of food and collation of record) May influence normal food intake Labour intensive to evaluate, therefore higher costs Subject requires literacy skills Long periods may reduce compliance/accuracy of record
Unweighed diet records	Less labour intensity than weighed dietary record Useful when quantification of food less important than meal patterns Good for assessing dietary balance Good for investigating relationships between food intake and symptoms/moods Can achieve information for a number of days Can also be used as a tool for treatment (highlights triggers to eating, dietary patterns, assessing compliance)	High workload for subject (collation of record) May influence normal food intake Labour intensive to evaluation, therefore higher costs Subject requires literacy skills Long periods may reduce compliance/accuracy of record
Checklist record	Reduces recall required as tick of foods as consumed Through computer systems analysis can be rapid	Checklist can be very long Foods may be missing Requires literacy but not as much as food records

Assessment of physical activity and exercise

Some useful definitions

Before commencing the physical activity assessment, it is important to become familiar with the terms 'physical activity' and 'exercise' (Box 4.6).

Box 4.6 Definitions

***Physical activity*:** is defined as any bodily movement that is produced by the contraction of skeletal muscle and that substantially increases energy expenditure.

***Physical fitness*:** is defined as a set of attributes that people have or achieve that relates to the ability to perform physical activity. The health-related components of physical fitness include the following: body composition, cardiovascular endurance, flexibility, muscular endurance, and muscular strength.

***Exercise*:** is a subclass of physical activity, defined as planned, structured, and repetitive bodily movement done to improve or maintain one or more components of physical fitness.

***Aerobic exercise*:** Exercise in which aerobic (oxidative) metabolism is used to generate the energy required to perform an activity. Regular aerobic exercise increases the functional capacity of the cardiovascular system. Characteristics of this type of exercise include:

- rhythmical movements of large muscle groups
- continuous and sustained.

Aerobic exercises include activities such as brisk walking, running, cycling, and swimming.

How much physical activity is enough?

The overall goal of the programme is to achieve the national recommendations for physical activity participation.

30 minutes of moderate-intensity activity on a minimum of 5 days of the week

However, in relation to physical activity and exercise in the management of CVD, particular benefit is observed with activities that result in gains in physical fitness, most typically through activities and structured exercise that are aerobic in nature, as summarized in Box 4.7. Therefore the preventive cardiology programme aims to achieve a more structured specific activity plan on at least three occasions of the week and on other days promotes the general recommendations of 30 minutes per day of moderate-intensity physical activity.

Box 4.7 The FITT principle associated with increased physical fitness

Frequency:	3–5 times per week
Intensity:	Moderate 60–80% heart rate maximum 12–14 Borg rating of perceived exertion scale (see Box 8.10)
Time:	15 minutes graduated warm-up 20–30 minutes conditioning 10 minutes cool-down
Type:	Cardiovascular Low skill

Assessment of physical activity, exercise and physical fitness

Physical activity behaviour is complicated and dynamic, resulting in challenges in its measurement. In recognition that there is no single variable that can reliably describe and predict physical activity, a preventive cardiology programme should include a number of physical activity measures to gain an insight into each individual's current physical activity participation, physical fitness, physical ability, perceptions, and beliefs of physical activity and degree of exposure to professional support and advice. Ultimately the aim of the assessment is to identify if the individual is achieving the levels of activity, as specified above, associated with reduced cardiovascular risk as well as the wider aspects that influence current and future participation.

Measurement of physical activity and exercise

Many methods are available to measure physical activity and exercise. The gold standard measure is 'doubly labelled water', but this is impractical in a clinical setting. Some examples for use in clinical settings include:

- Self-report methods, e.g. self-administered/interview-administered questionnaires.
- Motion sensors, e.g. pedometers and accelerometers.
- Aerobic capacity, e.g. maximal and sub-maximal exercise testing.
- Muscle strength and endurance, e.g. one repetition maximum, dynamometer.
- Flexibility, e.g. sit and reach test.
- Heart rate, e.g. resting, exercise, and recovery.
- Body composition, e.g. body mass index, bioelectric impedance, body folds.

Table 4.6 Advantages and limitations of physical activity and exercise measures

	Advantages	Limitations
• Self-report methods of physical activity, e.g. 7-day activity recall	• Easy to administer • Takes little time • Inexpensive • Low participant burden • Can estimate energy expenditure from daily living	• Reliability and validity problems associated with recall • Tendency for overestimation of activity • Suitability of questionnaires varies in different populations
• Accelerometers	• More objective indicator of body movement (accelerometers) • Provides indicator of intensity, frequency, and duration • Minute by minute information and can record data for periods of time (weeks) • Non-invasive	• Financial cost • Inaccurate assessment of a large range of activities (e.g. upper body, water-based activities • Cannot guarantee accurate placement of monitor
• Pedometers	• Inexpensive, non-invasive • Practical and easy in a number of settings • Potential to promote behaviour change	• Unable to detect intensity so loss of accuracy when jogging or running • Possibility of participant tampering • Pedometers limited to walking-based activity
• Aerobic capacity, e.g. cardiopulmonary exercise testing	• Objective • Valuable information for exercise prescription (e.g. prognosis, risk stratification for exercise training)	• Time consuming • Associated risk (maximal testing) • Not necessarily an indicator of low-level habitual activity • More invasive
• Muscle strength and endurance,	• Easy and simple to test	• Risk associated (1 repetition maximum) • Not necessarily an indicator of cardiorespiratory fitness

Table 4.6 Advantages and limitations of physical activity and exercise measures (*Continued*)

	Advantages	**Limitations**
• Flexibility	• Easy and simple • Inexpensive	• Not necessarily an indicator of cardiorespiratory fitness
• Heart rate	• Easy and simple • Inexpensive	• Modified by many extrinsic factors (e.g. temperature, caffeine, medications, etc.)
• Body composition	• Easy and simple to measure • Indirectly can indicate activity participation	• BMI does not take increased lean mass into consideration • Bioelectric impedance influenced by hydration status • Inhibitory factors in measurement of body folds

Assessment of physical activity and exercise in a preventive cardiology programme

A comprehensive assessment should include a selection of the measures highlighted above to capture physical activity and exercise status as well as consider other factors that impact on participation. One example of the content of a comprehensive physical activity assessment is presented in Table 4.7.

Table 4.7 A comprehensive physical activity assessment

Assessment	Example of measurement tool
Previous participation in physical activity and exercise	Self-report (e.g. questionnaire)
Current participation in physical activity and exercise	Self-report (e.g. activity log, 7-day activity recall, physical activity questionnaire) Motion sensor (e.g. pedometer)
Functional capacity, exercise responses	Submaximal exercise testing (e.g. cycle ergometer, step test, walk-based test protocols)
Functional limitations and physical restrictions	Body chart assessment of neurological or musculoskeletal dysfunctions Functional limitations questionnaire
Activity barriers and motivators, stage of behaviour change, exercise and activity, health beliefs	Self-report (e.g. questionnaire)
Risk stratification for exercise	American Association of Cardiovascular and Pulmonary Rehabilitation (AACVPR) tool for risk stratification

Self-report methods

- There are a number of well-established self-report methods for physical activity, ranging from activity logs to structured questionnaires. Common to the majority is the expression of the 'dose' of activity as a measure of energy expenditure. Activities can be 'scored' when the energy requirements of the activity are known. Energy required is calculated by frequency, intensity (expressed as METS), and duration of the mode of each activity reported.
- Mode (type)
- Frequency
- Intensity
- Duration

→

Activity level categorization
Energy expenditure

What is a MET?

The metabolic equivalent (MET) is typically used in exercising clinical populations as a means of expressing energy usage/expenditure. One metabolic equivalent (1 MET) is defined as the amount of energy required to serve the body's energy needs at rest (see Table 8.2 p. 159).

One MET equals an oxygen uptake (VO_2) of 3.5 ml/kg of body mass/minute (3.5 ml kg^{-1} min^{-1}). The energy requirement of an activity may be expressed as a multiple of one's resting metabolic rate. For example, walking at 4 mph requires an oxygen consumption five times that of the oxygen consumption to sit at rest (5 METs).

Using METs to score self-reported activity

When allocating a score to a self-report log, or alternatively the methods used within questionnaires, allocate a MET value based on the intensity of the activity reported, i.e. light, moderate, or vigorous:

- Sleep/rest = 1 MET
- Light = 1.5–2 METS
- Moderate = 3–7 METS
- Vigorous = 8+ METS.

With these values in mind, a weekly diary of sleep and activity can be converted as follows:

Sleep:	60.0 h × 1 MET = 60 kcal/kg
Light:	99.5 h × 1.5 METs = 149 kcal/kg
Moderate:	3.5 h × 4 METs = 14 kcal/kg
Vigorous:	2.5 h × 6 METs = 15 kcal/kg
Very vigorous:	2.5 h × 10 METs = 25 kcal/kg

Total weekly energy expenditure = 263 kcal/kg/week
Per day = 37.6 kcal/kg/day

If the body weight of the individual is known, energy expenditure can be expressed in absolute terms.

For example, for a 70-kg individual:
37.6 kcal/kg/day × 70 kg = 2632 kcal/day

In addition to these relative or absolute expressions of energy expenditure, categorization of activity status is also possible. There are many different examples, e.g. the Caspersen and Powell activity classification (Table 4.8).

Table 4.8 Caspersen and Powell activity classification

Sedentary	No leisure time physical activity
Irregularly active	Activity performed <3 times/week, <20 min bout, or both
Regularly active, not intensive	≥3 times/week, ≥20 min bout, and either <60% of maximum cardiovascular respiratory capacity[a]
Regularly active intensive	≥3 times/week, ≥20 min bout, and either ≥60% of maximum cardiovascular respiratory capacity[a] and involving dynamic activity of the large muscle groups

[a] Age and sex-specific estimates of maximum capacity:

Men: maximum capacity (METS) = [(60 – 0.55) × age (years)] ÷ 3.5

Women: maximum capacity (METS) = [(48 – 0.37) × age (years)] ÷ 3.5

60% maximum capacity = maximum capacity × 0.6.

Self-report methods: interview and self-administered questionnaires
Many questionnaires are available to measure physical activity and exercise. It is essential that the questionnaires selected are sensitive and can be generalized to the population being assessed. Some questionnaires focus on occupational activity and would therefore not be suitable for a retired older adult; others focus on leisure activity, which may underestimate activity in an older adult doing less structured activity and more activities of daily living, such as gardening. One commonly used questionnaire in cardiovascular disease prevention and rehabilitation in the UK is the Short Physical Activity Questionnaire (Box 4.8).

Box 4.8 The Short Physical Activity Questionnaire

1. Considering a 7-day period (a week), how many times on average do you do the following kinds of exercise for **more than 15 minutes** (write the appropriate number in the boxes)? *Record number of times.*

   a. **Strenuous activity (heart beats rapidly/tiring)?** (e.g. running, jogging, vigorous long-distance cycling, circuit training, aerobic dance, skipping, football, squash, basketball, roller skating, vigorous swimming) *No. of times* ❑

   b. **Moderate activity (not exhausting)?** (e.g. fast walking, mowing the lawn, tennis, easy cycling, badminton, easy swimming, ballroom dancing, fast or high step-ups) *No. of times* ❑

   c. **Mild activity (minimal effort)?** (e.g. easy walking, slow dancing, standing active fishing, bowling, golf, low step-ups) *No. of times* ❑

2. Considering a **7-day period** (a week), how often do you engage in any regular activity long enough to work up a sweat (heart beats rapidly)?
   Please tick Often ❑ Sometimes ❑ Never/Rarely ❑
3. Do you take regular physical activity of at least 30 minutes' duration on average 5 times a week? Yes ❑ No ❑

Rationale for including self-reported physical activity

- Self-reported measures of physical activity provide useful information in gaining an understanding of each individual's previous and current activity participation, as well as providing an insight into activities that are both enjoyable and of interest.
- By observation of activity over a period of a week (e.g. by an activity log or 7-day activity recall) the physical activity specialist can determine whether individuals are achieving the current recommended levels of 30 minutes of moderate-intensity activity on at least 5 days of the week.
- Activity logs can positively influence behaviour as individuals may become more aware of their activity levels.

Motion sensors (accelerometer, pedometer)

The gold standard would be the inclusion of accelerometer to validate self-reported activity and provide a more objective indicator of energy expenditure. However accelerometers are costly and hence the more affordable pedometer can be considered as a more limited but suitable alternative.

- Pedometers should only be used in individuals where walking is their main reported activity.
- The pedometer should be provided with a log sheet to record steps per day over a period of at least a week.
- Clear verbal and written instructions should be provided regarding placement and setting the pedometer each day.
- Pedometers can also be used to motivate behaviour and included as part of the intervention. Goals can include steps per day.

Exercise testing

Coronary patients entering a cardiovascular prevention and rehabilitation programme may have already been exposed to previous exercise testing procedures as part of their diagnostic investigations. These test results can be useful as part of the assessment process, although in reality the information gained can be limited, i.e. the test is often completed prior to subsequent interventions and often off medications. None the less, exercise capacity and exercise responses can provide useful information for risk stratification in exercise and exercise prescription planning.

Submaximal functional capacity testing

As part of a comprehensive preventive cardiology programme it is useful to assess functional capacity and exercise responses using a submaximal exercise test. There are many possible options and selection should be based on current ability, physical restrictions, and familiarity of activity (see Table 4.9).

Table 4.9 Submaximal tests for functional capacity in a preventive cardiology programme

	Examples	Brief description	Main advantages	Main limitations
Walk-based tests	6-minute walk test	• Non-incremental self-paced test over a 25 metre track • Metres per minute, heart rate and exertion level recorded for a 'comfortable' walking speed each minute for a period of 6 minutes • Score includes: total metres scored, average metres per minute, average MET score and number and length of rest periods where indicated	• Familiarity of activity • Particularly suitable for the low-capacity individual	• Unable to assess response to incremental workloads • Performance influenced by extrinsic factors (e.g. motivation)
	Incremental shuttle walk test (adapted)	• Designed originally for chronic obstructive pulmonary disease (COPD) patients • External pacing of incremental walking speeds around a 10 metre length • Score includes total metres scored, MET score and heart rate and exertion level for fixed submaximal workloads	• Familiarity of activity • Incremental and able to assess heart rate and exertion for increasing intensity • Assist in familiarizing the rating of perceived exertion scale	• Inherent warm-up period provided as initial speeds are very slow • 1-minute intervals and therefore unable to assess steady state

Step tests	Chester step test (adapted)	• External pacing of incremental stepping onto and off of a step of known height • Score includes total minutes achieved, METs score and heart rate and exertion level for fixed submaximal workloads	• Incremental and able to assess heart rate and exertion for increasing intensity • Assist in familiarizing the rating of perceived exertion scale • 2-minute increments so more likely to achieve steady-state responses	• Unsuitable for individuals with orthopaedic restrictions • Degree of co-ordination required
Cycle test	Monarch bike test	• Incremental workload at 2-minute intervals • Score includes total minutes achieved, METs score and heart rate and exertion level for fixed submaximal workloads	• Suitable for individuals with poor balance or restrictions in weight-bearing activities • Incremental and able to assess heart rate and exertion for increasing intensity • Assist in familiarizing the rating of perceived exertion scale • 2-minute increments so more likely to achieve steady-state responses	• Less familiar activity for some individuals • Unsuitable for individuals with reduced knee or hip range of movement • Degree of co-ordination required

Rationale for exercise testing in preventive cardiology programmes
- Diagnosis and prognosis
- Risk stratification for exertion-related events
- Future morbidity and mortality prediction
- Determine baseline fitness to evaluate changes in exercise capacity from training
- Guidance for physical activity and/or prescribing exercise training

Functional limitation and physical restrictions

A body chart method (Fig. 4.4) can be used to record any neurological or musculoskeletal dysfunctions. This is useful as during exercise it can provide a quick reference point for the need to adapt exercises or activities accordingly.

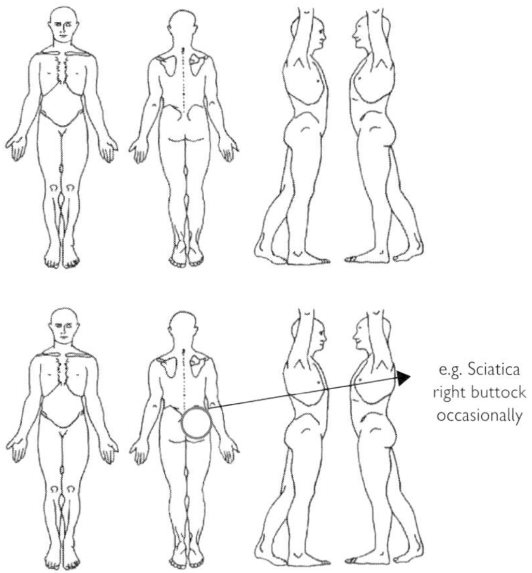

Fig. 4.4 In addition to reporting and assessment of physical restrictions, it is useful to assess functional limitation, using, for example, adapted questions from the SF-36 Questionnaire (Box 4.9). This provides a functional score that could reflect changes in quality of life over time.

Box 4.9 Functional Limitations Questionnaire (SF-36)

Functional limitations profile: The following items are about activities you might do during a typical day. Does your health *now* limit you in these activities? If so, how much?

Activities	Yes, limited a lot	Yes, limited a little	No, not limited at all
Vigorous activities: such as running, lifting heavy objects, participating in strenuous sports	1	2	3
Moderate activities: such as moving a table, pushing a vacuum cleaner, bowling, or playing golf	1	2	3
Lifting or carrying groceries	1	2	3
Climbing **several** flights of stairs	1	2	3
Climbing **one** flight of stairs	1	2	3
Bending, kneeling, or stooping	1	2	3
Walking **more than a mile**	1	2	3
Walking **more than ½ mile**	1	2	3
Walking **more than a ¼ mile**	1	2	3
Bathing or dressing yourself	1	2	3
TOTAL SCORE			

Activity barriers and motivators, stage of behaviour change, exercise, and activity health beliefs

It is essential to personalize the intervention, to be sensitive to the attitudes and beliefs of an individual towards activity.

Assessing stage of change will allow the subsequent intervention to be more specific and targeted, and more likely to be successful. Stage of change can be assessed by using specific questions.

Assessing stage of change for activity

Do you exercise regularly according to that definition?	
Yes, I have been for MORE than 6 months	= 1
Yes, I have been for LESS than 6 months	= 2
No, but I intend to in the next 30 days	= 3
No, but I intend to in the next 6 months	= 4
No, and I do NOT intend to in the next 6 months	= 5
Don't know/ Unsure	= 9

Another example includes the following:

Please read each of the statements below and then choose **one** statement that most clearly describes the individual:

Identify the statement the individual agrees with:

1. I currently do no moderate or vigorous activity and have no plans to do so in the next 6 months
2. I currently do no moderate or vigorous activity but plan to in the next 6 months though not in the next 30 days
3. Currently I do no moderate or vigorous activity but plan to in the next 6 months within the next 30 days
4. I currently participate in moderate or vigorous activities regularly (2–3 times a week). I started within the last 6 months
5. I currently participate in moderate or vigorous activities regularly (2– times a week). I started more than 6 months ago
6. I have participated in moderate or vigorous activities at some time in the past 6 months but have not done so recently.

STAGE OF CHANGE

1= Precontemplation	**2 = Contemplation**	**3 = Planning**
4 = Action	**5 = Maintenance**	**6 = Relapse**

Assessing the individual's view

What does the patient think about his/her current levels of physical activity / exercise? (tick one)

❑ Satisfied with their current levels

❑ Dissatisfied

❑ Not considered

Would the patient like to increase his/her levels of physical activity?

Yes / No / Unsure

Recording barriers to physical activity and exercise

Within the assessment the activities and exercise that are positively experienced, i.e. enjoyed by the individual or perhaps activities they have an interest to take up, should be noted. It is essential that activities that are not enjoyed should also be noted, as well as the individual's barriers to participating in physical activity and exercise. This information is vital to effective goal setting and prescription planning.

Risk stratification for exercise

Prior to participation in exercise training or providing an activity plan, the risk stratification for exercise should be completed. One common method used is the American Association of Cardiovascular and Pulmonary Rehabilitation (AACVPR) risk stratification for exercise tool (Table 4.10).

Screening partners and relatives

In a comprehensive programme, family members should be invited to participate fully and hence would undertake the same assessment procedures. As these individuals have not necessarily been referred through a medical route, in addition a Physical Activity Readiness Questionnaire (PAR-Q) (Box 4.10) should be completed.

Table 4.10 Risk stratification for exercise (AACVPR, 2004)

Lowest risk	Moderate risk	Highest risk
Absence of complex ventricular arrhythmias during exercise testing and recovery		Presence of complex ventricular arrhythmias during exercise testing or recovery
Absence of angina or other significant symptoms (e.g. unusual SOB, light-headedness or dizziness, during exercise testing and recovery)	Presence of angina or other significant symptoms (e.g. unusual shortness of breath (SOB), light-headedness or dizziness, occurring only at high levels of exertion (>7 METs))	Presence of angina or other significant symptoms (e.g. unusual SOB, light-headedness or dizziness at low levels of exertion (<5 METs) or during recovery)
	Mild to moderate level of silent ischaemia during exercise testing or recovery (ST-segment depression <2 mm from baseline)	High level of silent ischaemia (ST-segment depression >2 mm from baseline) during exercise testing or recovery
Presence of normal haemodynamic responses during exercise testing and recovery (appropriate increases and decreases in heart rate and systolic blood pressure (SBP) with increasing workloads and recovery)		Presence of abnormal haemodynamics with exercise testing (i.e. chronotropic incompetence or flat or decreasing SBP with increasing workloads) or recovery (severe postexercise hypotension)
		History of cardiac arrest, or sudden death

Functional capacity >7 METs	Functional capacity <5 METs	
Rest ejection fraction (EF) > 50%	Resting EF 40–49%	Rest EF < 40%
Uncomplicated myocardial infarction (MI) or revascularization procedure		Complicated MI or revascularization procedure
Absence of complicated ventricular arrhythmias at rest		Complex dysrhythmias at rest
Absence of congestive heart failure (CHF)		Presence of CHF
Absence of signs or symptoms of postevent/ postprocedure ischaemia		Presence of signs or symptoms of postevent/ postprocedure ischaemia
Absence of clinical depression		Presence of clinical depression
Lowest classification is assumed when each of the above factors in this category is present.	Moderate risk is assumed for patients who do not meet the classification of either highest or lowest.	Highest risk classification is assumed when the presence of any one of the above factors in this category is present.

Box 4.10 Physical Activity Readiness Questionnaire

Regular physical activity is fun and healthy, and increasingly more people are starting to become more active everyday. Being more active is very safe for most people. However, some people should check with their doctor before they start becoming much more physically active. If you are planning to become much more physically active than you are now, start by answering the seven questions in the box below. If you are between the ages of 15 and 69, the Par-Q will tell you if you should check with your doctor before you start. If you are over 69 years of age, and you are not used to being very active, check with your doctor. Common sense is your best guide when you answer these questions. Please read the questions carefully and answer each one honestly. Circle **Y for YES** or **N for NO**

1. **Has your doctor ever said that you have a heart condition and that you should only do physical activity recommended by a doctor?**
2. **Do you feel pain in your chest when you do physical activity?**
3. **In the past month, have you had chest pain when you were not doing physical activity?**
4. **Do you lose your balance because of dizziness or do you ever lose consciousness?**
5. **Do you have a bone or joint problem that could be made worse by a change in your physical activity?**
6. **Is your doctor currently prescribing drugs (for example, water pills) for your blood pressure or heart condition?**
7. **Do you know of any other reason why you should not do physical activity?**

If You Answered	YES to one or more questions
	Talk with your doctor by phone or in person **BEFORE** you start becoming much more physically active or **BEFORE** you have a fitness appraisal. Tell your doctor about the Par-Q and which questions you answered YES. • You may be able to do any activity you want – as long as you start slowly and build up gradually. Or, you may need to restrict your activities to those which are safe for you. Talk with your doctor about the kinds of activities you wish to participate in and follow his/her advice. • Find out which community programs are safe and helpful for you.

NO to all questions

If you answered NO honestly to all PAR-Q questions, you can be reasonably sure that you can:

- start becoming much more physically active – begin slowly and build up gradually. This is the safest and easiest way to go.
- Take part in a fitness appraisal – this is an excellent way to determine your basic fitness so that you can plan the best way for you to live actively.

DELAY BECOMING MUCH MORE ACTIVE• If you are not feeling well because of a temporary illness such as a cold or fever – wait until you feel better.• If you are or may be pregnant – talk to your doctor before you start becoming more active.

Please note: If your health changes so that you answer YES to any of the above questions, tell your fitness or health professional. Ask whether you should change your health activity plan.

I have read, understood and completed this questionnaire. Any questions I had were answered to my full satisfaction.

NAME____________________ **SIGNATURE**____________________ **DATE**___/___/_____

Assessment of other cardiovascular risk factors

Blood pressure

The large physiological variations in blood pressure (BP) mean that, blood pressure should be measured in each individual several times on several separate occasions:

- If systolic and/or diastolic blood pressure is only slightly elevated, repeated measurements should be made over a period of several months to achieve an acceptable definition of the individual's 'usual' blood pressure and to decide about initiating drug treatment.
- If systolic and/or diastolic blood pressure is more markedly elevated, repeated measurements are required within a shorter period of time (weeks or days) in order to make treatment decisions. This is also the case if there is an evidence of end-organ damage, and/or concomitance of other cardiovascular risk factors increasing overall cardiovascular risk.
- Raised BP requiring treatment should be confirmed during at least two to three visits, with a minimum of two BP readings taken per visit.

Box 4.11 Blood pressure measurement by conventional sphygmomanometer

- Use a properly maintained, calibrated, and validated device.
- Measure sitting blood pressure routinely; standing blood pressure should be recorded at the initial estimation in elderly and diabetic people to detect possible orthostatic hypotension.
- Blood pressure measurement is carried out from the right or the left arm, after the patient has rested for 5 min.
- Remove tight clothing, ensure hand relaxed, and avoid talking during the measurement procedure.
- Use cuff of appropriate size. Use a standard bladder (12–13 cm long and 35 cm wide) but have a larger bladder available for fat arms and a smaller one for thin arms.
- Have the cuff at the level of the heart, whatever the position of the patient.
- Deflate the cuff at a speed of 2 mmHg/s.
- Read blood pressure to the nearest 2 mmHg.
- Use phase I and V (disappearance) Korotkoff sounds to identify systolic (SBP) and diastolic (DBP) blood pressure, respectively.
- Measure BP in both arms at first visit to detect possible differences due to peripheral vascular disease. In this instance, take the higher value as the reference reading.
- Take the mean of at least two readings spaced by 1–2 min; more recordings are needed if marked differences between initial measurements are found.
- Do not treat on the basis of an isolated reading.

Devices measuring blood pressure in the fingers or on the wrist should be avoided because of possible inaccuracy.

Table 4.11 Definition and classification of blood pressure levels[7]

Category	Systolic (mmHg)		Diastolic (mmHg)
Optimal	<120	and	<80
Normal	120–129	and/or	80–84
High normal	130–139	and/or	85–89
Grade 1 hypertension	140–159	and/or	90–99
Grade 2 hypertension	160–179	and/or	100–109
Grade 3 hypertension	≥180	and/or	≥110
Isolated systolic hypertension	≥140	and	<90

Isolated systolic hypertension should be graded (1, 2, 3) according to systolic blood pressure values in the ranges indicated, provided that diastolic values are <90 mmHg. Grades 1, 2, and 3 correspond to classification of mild, moderate, and severe hypertension, respectively. These terms have now been omitted to avoid confusion with quantification of total cardiovascular risk (© ESC 2007).

7 Graham, I., Atar, D., Borch-Johnsen, K. *et al.* (2007). European guidelines on cardiovascular disease prevention in clinical practice: full text. Fourth Joint Task Force of the European Society of Cardiology and other Societies on Cardiovascular Disease Prevention in Clinical Practice. *European Journal of Cardiovascular Prevention and Rehabilitation*, **14**(Suppl 2), S1–S113.

Measurement of lipids

What and when?

Total cholesterol and HDL can usually be measured in a non-fasting state. In patients who are found to be at high risk, however, a full lipid profile including total cholesterol (TC), low-density lipoprotein cholesterol (LDL-C), high-density lipoprotein cholesterol (HDL-C), and triglycerides (TG) is recommended.

LDL-cholesterol is usually not directly measured but is calculated from the other lipid values according to the Friedewald formula.[8]

Friedewald formula

LDL-cholesterol = Total cholesterol – HDL cholesterol – (TG/2.2)

Note

- This method cannot accurately be applied in the non-fasting state as post-prandial rises in triglyceride levels are common.
- It also cannot be used if fasting triglycerides >4 mmol/\l.
- Ideally therefore, a full lipid profile should be done after a 12-hour fast.

To avoid lack of standardization, lipid analyses should be performed in a laboratory with recognized quality assurance.

Post-myocardial infarction

In patients who have had a myocardial infarction, it is recommended that lipid levels are estimated within the first 24 hours of their event, as after this period they become gradually lower than the patient's premorbid levels for an average of 6–8 weeks.[9]

Other factors affecting lipid levels

Biological variation

- Occurs for many reasons, including diurnal variation, seasonal variation, diet, smoking, and physical activity levels.
- Can result in significant variation in intra-individual serum lipid values—approximately 6.0% for TC, 7.0% for HDL, 10% for LDL-C, and 23.0% for triglycerides.[10]
- Measuring sequential lipid profiles, e.g. a week apart, may help reduce biological variation, but is often not clinically practical.

Alcohol

- Intake prior to blood collection may temporarily elevate TG levels.
- Prolonged moderate intake may result in an elevated HDL-C serum level.[10]

Diabetes

- Poorly controlled diabetes can be associated with low HDL-C levels, small dense LDL-C particles (pro-atherogenic) and higher triglyceride levels[11]
- Improving glycaemic control can reverse these changes.

Thyroid disease

- In hypothyroidism, total cholesterol, HDL-C, and LDL-C are predominantly increased with only a slight increase in triglycerides.
- Hyperthyroidism has an opposite effect.[12]

Always check thyroid function when initially measuring lipids.

8 Friedewald, W.T., Levy, R.I., and Fredrickson, D.S. (1972). Estimation of the concentration of low-density lipoprotein cholesterol in plasma, without use of the preparative ultracentrifuge. *Clinical Chemistry*, **18**(6), 499–502.

9 Fyfe, T., Baxter, R.H., Cochran, K.M., and Booth, E.M. (1971). Plasma-lipid changes after myocardial infarction. *Lancet*, **2**(7732), 997–1001.

10 Cooper, G.R., Myers, G.L., Smith, S.J., and Schlant, R.C. (1992). Blood lipid measurements. Variations and practical utility. *Journal of the American Medical Association*, **267**(12), 1652–60.

11 Nesto, R.W. (2005). Beyond low-density lipoprotein: addressing the atherogenic lipid triad in type 2 diabetes mellitus and the metabolic syndrome. *American Journal of Cardiovascular Drugs*, **5**(6), 379–87.

12 Friis, T. and Pedersen, L.R. (1987). Serum lipids in hyper- and hypothyroidism before and after treatment. *Clinica Chimica Acta*, **162**(2), 155–63.

Dysglycaemia

Why assess blood glucose (glycaemia)?

- Blood glucose has a continuous relationship with CVD risk, similar to that of blood pressure and cholesterol in those without diabetes.
- This risk is influenced by other risk factors, such as smoking, and thus assessment of blood glucose is important in a cardiovascular risk assessment.
- Individuals with diabetes have a two- to fourfold increase in the relative risk of CVD.
- In those with acute coronary syndromes, approximately one-quarter to one-third of patients without previously known diabetes will have evidence of dysglycaemia.

How is dysglycaemia diagnosed?

The gold standard diagnosis is the oral glucose tolerance test (OGTT), which usually consists of the oral administration of a 75 g glucose load with measurement of plasma glucose 2 hours later. Dysglycaemia may be classified into the following three categories (Table 4.12):

- Impaired fasting glycaemia (IFG)
- Impaired glucose tolerance (IGT)
- Diabetes mellitus.

An OGTT is the gold standard diagnostic test for the following reasons:

- Fasting plasma glucose alone fails to diagnose ~30% of cases of diabetes.
- It is the only way of diagnosing IGT, which is itself associated with an increased cardiovascular risk of ~1.5 compared to those with normal glucose tolerance.

Measuring glycated haemoglobin ($HbA1_c$)

Glycated haemoglobin reflects the average level of glucose to which the red blood cell has been exposed during its life cycle (4 weeks to 3 months).

While $HbA1_c$ should not be used to diagnose diabetes, its measurement will assess diabetes control and effectiveness of therapy over this time period.

Good glycaemic control has been shown equivocally to reduce the incidence of microvascular complications in both type 1 and type 2 diabetes. It is also likely to reduce the incidence of macrovascular complications.

Optimal management targets are a normal $HbA1_c$ (<6.0%). In clinical practice, a more practical target is ≤6.5% (JBS2/International Diabetes Federation/European Society of Diabetes).

Table 4.12 World Health Organization diagnostic criteria for diabetes (2006)

	Normal	IFG	IGT	Diabetes
Fasting plasma glucose (mmol/l)	<6.0	>6.1 and <7.0	OGTT required to diagnose	>7.0
2 h post 75 g oral glucose load (mmol/l)	<7.8	<7.8	≥7.8 and <11.1	≥11.1

Assessment of psychological and social factors

The concept of psychological and social health recognizes the contribution of the social, cultural, environmental, and psychological aspects of a person and their microenvironment (family and community) to their health, to the onset of illness, to both health and illness behavior, and often the prognosis of an illness

Elements of psychosocial health

- Health Status and Health Related Quality of Life (HRQoL).
- Beliefs and perceptions about illness.
- Risk perception.
- Social and family status.

Why measure psychosocial health?

Clinical

- To provide a context to the assessment of lifestyle and CVD risk factors that creates a holistic view of the patient in his or her environment.
- To screen for psychological morbidity.
- To gain an understanding of beliefs and misconceptions.
- To place the patient and his or her family in a socio-economic context.

These findings facilitate a tailoring of the programme to the individual requirements of each patient and family

Research

- To measure the impact of a programme from the patient's perspective.
- To improve patient outcomes: symptoms, mortality, satisfaction with care, function, and quality of life.

How to measure psychosocial health

- Validated tools.
- Self-administered questionnaires.
- Collection of information on social factors.

Health Related Quality of Life (HRQoL)

This is a patient-assessed health outcome measure which attempts to give health professionals and researchers an understanding of the patient's perspective of outcome, so that these outcomes can be improved.[13–15]

There are four main components of quality of life:

- Physical and occupational functioning
- Psychological state
- Social interaction
- Somatic sensation (symptoms).

The different tools to measure HRQoL can be classified as follows (see Fig. 4.5):

- Generic
- Disease or population specific
- Dimension specific
- Individualized
- Utility

A valid and reliable tool should be selected which is responsive to change and appropriate for the patient group. A tool which is not sensitive to change would not pick up on the benefits of programme attendance.

Choosing the right tool to measure HRQoL

- Look at the tools that are available before creating new ones.
- Generic tools can be used in any patient population. No single score is produced but summary scores for different categories. For example, the SF-36 has eight subscales which produce two summary scores.
- Utility questionnaires produce a health status score which can contribute to a health economics analysis.
- Using standardized instruments contributes to more meaningful service evaluation, so it is important to use tools that may feed into an audit process in your country. An example of such a process is the National Audit for Cardiac Rehabilitation (NACR) in the UK.
- HRQoL evaluation may be used to determine the best use of health care resources (value for money).

13 Garratt, A., Schmidt, L., Mackintosh, A., and Fitzpatrick, R. (2002). Quality of Life measurement: bibliographic study of patient assessed health outcome measures. *British Medical Journal*, **324**, 1417.

14 Hevey, D., McGee, H., and Horgan, J. (2004). Responsiveness of Health related Quality of Life Outcome measures in cardiac rehabilitation: comparison of cardiac rehabilitation outcome measures. *Journal of Clinical and Consulting Psychology*, **72**(6), 1175–80.

15 McGee, H. (2004). Quality of life. In A. Kaptein and J. Weinman (eds), *Health psychology*, (1st edn), pp. 234–57. Oxford: Blackwell Publishing.

Generic
- SF-36 (1992) and SF-12
- Dartmouth Co-op (1987)
- Nottingham Health Profile (1985)
- Duke Health Profile
- (1990)WHOQOL – 100 (1995)

Disease specific
- Canadian Cardiovascular Society angina disability scale (1976)
- The MacNew Heart Disease Questionnaire (1993)
- The Seattle Angina Questionnaire (1994)
- Minnesota Living with Heart Failure Questionnaire (1987)
- HeartQol (under development)

Dimension specific
- Cardiac Depression Scale (1996)
- Heart Patients' Psychological Questionnaire (1986)
- HADS (1983)
- Global Mood Scale (1993)
- Type D personality scale(1998)
- DASI (1989)

Individualized
- Schedule for the Evaluation of Individual Quality of Life (1991)
- Quality of Life Index (1985)

Utility
- EuroQol (EQ-5D) (1996)
- Quality of Wellbeing Scale (1993)

Fig. 4.5 Some examples of tools used to measure HRQoL.

Box 4.12 Appropriate characteristics of HRQoL instruments
- Is it user friendly?
- Validity (does it measure what it speaks to measure?)
- Reliability (are the measurements precise and reproducible?)
- Does it provide clinically significant information?
- Is it responsive to change over time?
- Does it provide an effective clinical screening tool?

A proposed package for measuring HRQoL (tools employed in the EUROACTION study)
- SF-36 (Functional Limitation Questions)
- Hospital Anxiety and Depression Scale (HADS)
- Global Mood Scale (positive dimensions)
- EQ-5D (utility measure)

These tools capture the multidimensional nature of HRQoL relevant to the priority groups of people that the preventive cardiology programme manages. In addition the EQ-5D facilitates a health economics analysis of the programme.

Use of the SF-36 Functional Limitation Questions is explained in Box 4.9.

Hospital Anxiety and Depression Scale (HADS)

Screening for anxiety and depression is important as both may affect adherence to treatment regimens. In addition, depression is an important predictor of mortality in coronary patients.

- Contains two subscales: anxiety and depression.
- The HADS is an example of a dimension-specific measure of HRQoL.
- Short and extensively validated.
- This tool is popular with both patients and health professionals.
- Translated and validated in several languages.

The questionnaire is divided equally between depression and anxiety items, although these items are mixed up within the questionnaire. The respondent ticks the appropriate response for him/her to each item. Anxiety and depression items are scored separately, thus producing two summary scores. The ranges in Table 4.13 give an idea of the level of anxiety and depression.

Table 4.13 Ranges for anxiety and depression scores using the HADS

Anxiety	**Depression**
Items with odd numbers (1, 3, 5, etc.)	Items with even numbers (2, 4, 6, etc.)
0–7 = Normal	0–7 = Normal
8–10 = Borderline abnormal	8–10 = Borderline abnormal
11–21 = Abnormal	11–21 = Abnormal

A score of 11 or more in either subscale should be the cut-off for onward referral for specialist help. The HADS provides a clinically meaningful psychological screening tool for patients, although it should not be used as a diagnostic tool.

The HADS is copyrighted. In order to purchase it and use it, it is necessary to seek permission, e-mail: international@nfer-nelson.co.uk

Global Mood Scale (GMS)

- The GMS was originally developed for use in cardiac patients and provides us with a validated scale that measures subjective moods and feelings.
- Affective mood status has been found to be a major dimension of HRQoL in cardiovascular patients.
- The GMS comprises 10 negative and 10 positive commonly reported mood terms.
- The positive affect subscale of the GMS has been shown to be the most responsive to change in cardiac rehabilitation.
- In the EUROACTION study the positive affect subscale was employed to assess the positive effect of the programme (see Table 4.14). A higher score (maximum 40) is associated with improved wellbeing.

- The GMS positive affect subscale is closely associated with overall quality of life, and higher scores on this subscale may be associated with enhanced emotional wellbeing in the future.

Table 4.14 Global Mood Scale

Below are a number of words that describe feelings and emotions. Please read **each item** carefully and then **mark the appropriate box** next to that word. Indicate to what extent **you have felt this way lately**. Please use the following scale to record your answers.

To what extent have you felt this way lately	Not at all	A little bit	Moderately	Quite a bit	Extremely
Active	0	1	2	3	4
Dynamic	0	1	2	3	4
Bright	0	1	2	3	4
Hard-working	0	1	2	3	4
Lively	0	1	2	3	4
Enterprising	0	1	2	3	4
Relaxed	0	1	2	3	4
Sociable	0	1	2	3	4
Cheerful	0	1	2	3	4
Self-confident	0	1	2	3	4

EQ-5D (EUROQOL)

- The EQ-5D is a standardized measure of health status and an example of a utility measure. Utility measures have been developed to facilitate a health economics appraisal of health interventions. These measures aim to assess the value of interventions in terms of a combination of quality of life and length of life (QALYs—quality-adjusted life years).
- The EQ-5D is applicable to a wide range of health conditions and treatments and is easy and fast to complete.
- It consists of two pages—the EQ-5D descriptive system and the EQ visual analogue scale (EQ VAS).
- The EQ-5D descriptive system identifies the level of problems (if any) via the responses to five questions representing five dimensions, which generates a weighted index (see Box 4.13).
- Respondents rate their health status using the EQ VAS, which is a visual analogue scale ranging from 0, which is the worst imaginable health state, to 100, which is the best imaginable health state (to analyse changes in health status over time).

Box 4.13 Five dimensions of the EQ-5D descriptive system

Mobility

Self-care

Usual activiteis

Pain/discomfort

Anxiety/depression

Permission to use the EQ-5D should be sought from the EuroQol group (www.euroqol.org) which is an international network of multidisciplinary researchers.

Using a generic multi-dimensional tool to measure HRQoL: a comparison of the SF-36 and the Dartmouth Co-op

Generic assessment tools can be used in any patient or population group. They usually contain several subscales and do not produce a single score.

Short Form 36 (SF-36)

- Developed from the American Medical Outcomes Study in 1992.
- A second version (SF36II) has been introduced by the Third Oxford Health and Lifestyles Study.
- Most widely used HRQoL instrument internationally.
- Comprehensive 36-item questionnaire with eight subscales, which produce two summary scores (Box 4.14).
- Translated and validated in several languages.
- Sensitive to low levels of disability.
- Useful in monitoring general and specific populations, comparing the burden of different diseases, differentiating the health benefits produced by different treatments, and in screening individual patients.

Box 4.14 SF-36 subscales

Subscale	Summary
Physical functioning	Physical health
Role physical	Physical health
Bodily pain	Physical health
General health	Physical health
Role emotional	Mental health
Social functioning	Mental health
Mental health	Mental health
Energy/vitality	Mental health

Permission and payment are required to use the SF-36 (www.sf-36.com). A shorter version of this tool is also available (SF-12).

Dartmouth Co-op

- Designed principally for use in everyday clinical practice.
- Provides a short and comprehensive survey of health status (30–45 seconds to complete each item).
- Nine items (Box 4.15).
- Each dimension has a possible score between 1 and 5 (see Fig. 4.6 for one example). The higher the score, the higher the level of disability.
- High levels of test–retest reliability.
- Compares well with longer measures (SF-36).
- Normative data are available for UK.

Box 4.15 Dartmouth Co-op assessment tool

Physical fitness	
Feelings	Change in health
Daily activities	Overall health
Social activities	Social support
Pain	Quality of life

FEELINGS

During the past 4 weeks . . .
How much have you been bothered by emotional problems such as feeling anxious, depressed, irritable or downhearted and blue?

Not at all		1
Slightly		2
Moderately		3
Quite a bit		4
Extremely		5

SUPPORT PROVIDED BY THE HENRY J. KAISER FAMILY FOUNDATION

Fig. 4.6 Dartmouth Co-op, scoring Feelings. The charts are available from: deborah.johnson@dartmouth.edu (http://www.dartmouth.edu/~coopproj/)

Table 4.15 Some practical considerations in choosing tool to measure HRQoL in people attending preventive cardiology programmes

Considerations	SF-36	Dartmouth coop	HADS	GMS	EQ-5D
Easy to complete and score		✓	✓	✓	✓
Widely validated	✓		✓		✓
Practical for a clinical setting		✓	✓		
Applicable to a wide range of conditions and treatments	✓	✓	✓	✓	✓
Sensitive to change	✓	✓	✓	✓	✓
Produces a utility score					✓
Validated translations available	✓		✓		✓
Sensitive to low levels of disability, mild symptoms	✓		✓		
Requires permission to use	✓		✓		✓
Requires payment to use	✓		✓		
Covers a broad range of HRQoL dimensions	✓	✓			✓
Test and retest reliability	✓	✓	✓		

Perceptions about illness

People who are diagnosed with a medical condition and their close family members may have irrational fears and misconceptions about their illness. These perceptions can influence:

- Emotions—causing distress, provoking guilt, inducing low self-esteem, and poor psychological adjustment.
- The adoption of health protective behaviours.
- Compliance with treatment.

Mismanagement of these fears and misconceptions may lead to:

- The adoption of passive coping strategies, such as avoidance and denial.
- Unnecessary dependence on health professionals.

Beliefs and perceptions about illness are activated by symptoms, diagnosis, and risk perception. They can be classified as follows:

- Identity or label of a diagnosis
- Cause
- Timeline
- Consequences
- Cure
- Control

Assessing these cognitions in patients and family members who are recruited to the programme will facilitate an understanding of the beliefs, perceptions and possible misconceptions that they may have of their illness, and will allow the programme to be tailored so as to improve adaptation to illness. For example, higher controllability beliefs are associated with more active coping with an illness and positive psychological adjustment.

The Illness Perception Questionnaire (IPQ-R)[16]

- This questionnaire provides a means of assessing the several different components of illness cognition (Box 4.15).
- In responding to the questionnaire, patients are able to express their coherent view of their illness by expressing their beliefs about each of the components.
- The following website has more information about the questionnaire: www.uib.no/ipq/.
- The EUROACTION project developed two versions of the questionnaire—one for use with patients with coronary artery disease and one for use with their partners. In Box 4.16 you can see how the items of the questionnaire were adopted to accommodate family members.
- These versions of the questionnaire allow not only the patient with a condition, but also their partners, to express their views about the illness and thus have a family context of illness cognition.

16 Moss-Morris, R., Weinman, J. *et al.* (2002). The revised Illness Perception Questionnaire (IPQ-R). *Psychology and Health*, **17**, 1–16.

Box 4.16 Components of illness representations

- **Timeline acute/chronic subscale**
  1. 'My illness will last for a long time'
  2. 'Heart disease will last for a long time'
- **Timeline cyclical subscale**
  1. 'My symptoms come and go in cycles'
  2. 'Heart disease symptoms…'
- **Consequences subscale**
  1. 'My illness has major consequences on my life'
  2. 'Heart disease has major consequences on a person's life'
- **Personal control subscale**
  1. 'Nothing I do will affect my illness'
  2. 'Nothing a person does will affect their heart disease'
- **Treatment control subscale**
  1. 'My treatment can control my illness'
  2. 'Treatment can control heart disease'
- **Illness coherence subscale**
  1. 'My illness is a mystery to me/I don't understand my illness'
  2. 'Heart disease is a mystery to me/I don't understand heart disease'
- **Emotional representations subscale**
  1. 'When I think about my illness I get upset'
  2. 'When I think about having heart disease I get upset'
- **Psychological attributes subscale**
  1. 'Worries or family problems caused my illness'
  2. 'Worry or family problems could cause heart disease for me'
- **Risk factors subscale**
  1. 'My illness is hereditary—it runs in my family'
  2. 'I could have heart disease because it is hereditary—it runs in my family'

  1. 'My illness is because of my diet or eating habits'
  2. 'I could have heart disease because of my diet or eating habits'

  1. 'My illness is because of smoking'
  2. 'I could have heart disease because of smoking'

  1. 'My illness is because of drinking alcohol'
  2. 'I could have heart disease because of drinking alcohol'
- **Immunity subscale**
  1. 'My illness is because of a germ or virus'
  2. 'I could have heart disease because of a germ or virus'
- **Accident or chance subscale**
  1. 'My illness is because of chance or bad luck'
  2. 'I could have heart disease because of chance or bad luck'

  1. -Patient version
  2. -Family member version

Risk perception

Risk perception incorporates beliefs about the susceptibility an individual has to develop health problems.

- Risk perception is positively associated with the use of health protective behaviours.
- Measuring risk perception can help professionals to tailor interventions to the individual:
  - for example, to use motivational techniques with those patients who are low risk perceivers
  - and to provide reassurance and reinforcement of the benefits of health protective action to those with high perceptions of risk.
- Moods and emotions can affect risk perception, with sad moods and worry leading to increased perceptions of risk, which may be irrational.
- The IPQ-R includes some questions on risk perception.
- For individuals at high risk of developing cardiovascular disease, the EUROACTION study employed risk perception questions based on the Danish Inter-99 study (Figs 4.7 and 4.8).
- The questionnaires were completed by both the patient and their partner, thus providing a family context of risk perception.

More information about these versions of the IPQ-R and risk perception questionnaires is available from the EUROACTION group (email: c.jennings@imperial.ac.uk). Translations are available in some European languages.

Risk perception — Initial Assessment

	Strongly disagree	Disagree	Neutral	Agree	Strongly agree
1a) In my opinion, everyone ought to know their risk of heart disease in order to reduce it					
1b) I am worried that I may develop heart disease					
1c) I am worried about finding out my risk of heart disease					

Your current habits

	No—not important	No—would not do	Not sure	Yes—probably	Yes—definitely
2) What do you plan to do to improve your own general health in the coming year?					
a. avoid stress					
b. stop smoking					
c. lose weight					
d. become more physically active					
e. eat a diet with less fat					
f. eat a diet with less cholesterol					
g. avoid sugar and sweets					
h. reduce my salt intake					
i. reduce my alcohol intake					
j. improve my job/work situation					
k. reduce my working hours					
l. have a more regular life routine					
m. get more sleep					
n. attend medical examinations more often					

Your health beliefs

	No—not important	No—would not do	Not sure	Yes—probably	Yes—definitely
3) What do you believe would reduce YOUR risk of getting a heart attack?					
a. avoid stress					
b. avoiding smoking					
c. avoiding being overweight					
d. being physically active					
e. eat a diet with less fat					
f. eat a diet with less cholesterol					
g. avoiding sugar and sweets					
h. reducing my salt intake					
i. reducing my alcohol intake					
j. ensuring I have a reasonable job/work situation					
k. ensuring I have reasonable working hours					
l. ensuring I have aregular life routine					
m. get enough sleep					
n. attending regular medical examinations					

4) What do you think your risk of getting heart disease is in the next 10 years?
B5

Very high	High	Moderate	Low	Very Low	Don't know

5) Do you think your risk of getting heart disease in the next 10 years is higher, lower or about the same as a person of the same age and sex as you?
B6

Much higher	Higher	About the same	Lower	Much lower

Fig. 4.7 Risk perception questionnaires (initial assessment).

Risk perception — End of Programme/one year

1) What did you do in the last year to improve your own health?	√
a. nothing in particular	
b. avoided stress	
c. stopped smoking	
d. lost weight	
e. became more physically active	
f. ate a diet with less fat	
g. ate a diet with less cholesterol	
h. ate a diet with less salt	
i. ate less sugar and sweets	
j. reduced my alcohol intake	
k. improved my work/job situation environment	
l. reduced my working hours	
m. had a more regular life routine	
n. got more sleep	
o. attended medical examinations more often	
p. other (explain)	

2) What do you think your risk of getting heart disease is in the next 10 years?

Very high	High	Moderate	Low	Very Low	Don't know

3) Do you think your risk of getting heart disease in the next 10 years is higher, lower or about the same as a person of the same age and sex as you?

Much higher	Higher	About the same	Lower	Much lower

4) Attitudes to health screening:	Strongly disagree	Disagree	Neutral	Agree	Strongly agree
a) I was satisfied with the way the nurse explained my risk of developing heart disease					
b) My quality of life has been reduced explained my risk of developing heart disease					
c) It was unpleasant to learn my risk of heart disease					
d) I wish I didn't know my risk of heart disease					
e) I was satisfied with getting to know my risk of heart disease—now I can act					
f) I am anxious about the future now that I have learned about my risk of heart disease					
g) In my view, my risk of getting heart disease is similar compared to other people of my age					

Fig. 4.8 Risk perception questionnaires (end of programme review and 1 year).

Social factors

- Low socio-economic status is an indicator of higher risk for cardiovascular disease. This is because more people with lower socio-economic status develop and die from cardiovascular disease, because of a clustering of risk factors including psychosocial, lifestyle, and biological factors.
- Psychosocial risk factors contribute independently to the risk of coronary disease and worsen the clinical course and prognosis.
- These risk factors include inadequate social support or lack of social networks, work stress, and depression. They are strongly linked with low socio-economic status, age, and gender, and are often associated with lifestyle and biological risk factors.
- Health behaviours can be stimulated by the support of a spouse, or other members of the household: for example, taking medications, stopping smoking, becoming physically active, eating healthily. The social support acts as an indirect mediator.

Indicators of social status

- Age/gender
- Marital status
- Living alone
- Perceived social support
- Socio-economic status (post code, education, occupation, retirement)
- Return to work (employment status)
- Ethnicity

Questions assessing social support

From Dartmouth Co-op

During the past week was someone available to help you if you needed and wanted help? For example:

		Reply options. (Enter a number in each box)
I. If you felt nervous, lonely, or blue	❑	1. Yes as much as I wanted
II. Got sick and had to stay in bed	❑	2. Yes quite a bit
III. Needed someone to talk to	❑	3. Yes some
IV. Needed help with daily chores	❑	4. Yes a little
V. Needed help with taking care of yourself	❑	5. No not at all

From the Enhancing Recovery in Coronary Heart Disease (ENRICHD) study
ESSI (ENRICHD Social Support Instrument)[17]

Item1	Is there someone available to whom you can count on to listen to you when you need to talk ?				
	None of the time ❑	A little of the time ❑	Some of the time ❑	Most of the time ❑	All of the time ❑
Item 2	Is there someone available to you to give you good advice about a problem ?				
Item 3	Is there someone available to you who shows you love and affection ?				
Item 4	Is there someone available to help with daily chores?				
Item 5	Can you count on anyone to provide you with emotional support (talking over problems or helping you make a difficult decision)?				
Item 6	Do you have as much contact as you would like with someone you feel close to, someone in whom you can trust and confide in?				
Item 7	Are you currently married or living with a partner ?				
	Yes ❑		No ❑		

17 Vaglio, J. *et al.* (2004). Testing the performance of the ENRICHD social support instrument in cardiac patients. *Health and Quality of Life Outcomes*, **2,** 24.

Family history of coronary heart disease

Family history and increased risk of heart disease

Individuals with a family history of coronary heart disease (CHD) are themselves at higher risk of developing heart disease (by a factor of ~ 1.5).

The definition of family history is generally accepted as referring to all first-degree relatives (parents, siblings and offspring).

This increased risk is independent of other risk factors associated with CHD such as obesity, raised blood pressure, lipid abnormalities, and impaired glucose regulation, which aggregate in families with CHD.

The age at which the parent had their event seems to be important

- an age <60 years conferring greater risk
- maternal history conferring higher risk

These characteristics support a polygenic type of inheritance for CHD with the timing of occurrence of clinical disease dependent on other factors such as smoking.

Assessing family history

Thus individuals with a family history of premature CHD are an important priority group for cardiovascular disease prevention. Whilst assessing family history, the following caveats should be borne in mind

- prone to information bias e.g. those with more relatives will be more likely to be classified as having a strong family history.
- knowledge amongst individuals with regards to their family history may vary in accuracy

Screening and follow up of first degree relatives of first degree relatives

Definition of premature atherosclerotic disease

- Men who present with symptomatic disease before the age of 55.
- Women who present with symptomatic disease before the age of 65.

First degree relatives of patients presenting with premature atherosclerotic disease:

- Sibling (brother or sister)
- Offspring (son or daughter)

What should the follow up of first degree relatives include?

- An assessment of lifestyle – smoking, diet and physical activity
- Risk factor screening - overweight and obesity, blood pressure, lipids and glucose
- Screening for familial dyslipidaemias
- A family history of premature CHD, or other atherosclerotic disease, should be taken into account in assessing the total risk of developing

CVD in a healthy individual, including taking of detailed history and drawing of a pedigree.

- Lifestyle advice and, where appropriate therapeutic management of risk factors should be offered to families where coronary disease is highly prevalent.
- Specialist care provided through a lipid clinic in those families affected by familial dyspipidaemias.

Responsibilities of the preventive cardiology programme team

- Identify all the first degree relatives of patients who present with premature disease
- Inform patients that these relatives should be followed up by their general practitioner or other family physician

Key references

Thomas, CB., Cohen, BH. The familial occurrence of hypertension and coronary artery disease, with observations concerning obesity and diabetes. Ann Intern Med 1955 January;42(1): 90-127.

Myers, RH., Kiely, DK., Cupples, LA., Kannel, WB. Parental history is an independent risk factor for coronary artery disease: the Framingham Study. Am Heart J 1990 October;120(4):963-9.

Hunt, SC., Williams, RR., Barlow, GK. A comparison of positive family history definitions for defining risk of future disease. J Chronic Dis 1986;39(10):809-21.

Part 2

Application of the assessment findings to manage lifestyle and cardiovascular risk factors

Chapter 5

Changing lifestyles

Changing lifestyles

Healthy choices should be easy choices. Making this a reality is achieved through healthy public policy and health education with a philosophy of personal empowerment at its base.

With this in mind—how can health professionals influence the choices their patients and families make?

Think about how you approach your patients . . .

- ***The medical model of prevention***—overmedicalizes patients and encourages the adoption of the sick role, discourages self-management, and can lead to labelling of people who choose not to comply with advice.
- ***The empowerment model***—gives people the genuine potential to make choices, raises critical awareness of the political, economic, and social issues relating to health, and it develops a high level of realistic self-esteem and life skills.

Box 5.1 Be aware of the power you hold

As health professionals we are valued for our expertise.
Take care to use this power in a constructive way:

DON'T	***DO***
• Force	• Allow choice
• Indoctrinate	• Raise critical awareness
• Use coercion	• Be facilitative
• Manipulate	• Share agenda setting
• Use hidden threats	• Be honest
• Be dictatorial	• Negotiate

Before embarking on helping patients and their families to adopt healthy lifestyle habits such as:

- Stopping smoking
- Eating cardio-protective foods
- Becoming more physically active
- Taking exercise
- Losing weight

. . . look at the factors that may be determining their health behaviour, such as:

- ***Social pressure*** —for example, family and friends' smoking and cooking habits.
- ***Social isolation***—there is no-one to reinforce the messages you give and to provide encouragement and support.
- ***Psychological need***—for example, unhealthy habits such as smoking may be perceived as being one of the only comforts in life, a way of coping with stress at work and in general.
- ***Social conditioning***—lifestyle habits may be seen as the social or religious norm.

- ***Socio-economic status***—cardiovascular risk factors are more prevalent in manual compared to non-manual workers and in those with a lower educational attainment. Healthy foods can be costly.
- ***Impaired health status***—for example, functional limitations in relation to exercise, anxiety, and depression.
- ***Health service provision***—for example, having cardiovascular disease prevention programmes in primary care.
- ***Legislation***—for example, bans on smoking in public places, provision of footpaths, cycle paths, and public leisure facilities.

Symptoms, diagnosis, and perceptions of risk can affect the beliefs a patient has about his or her illness and how amenable it is to control.

This may affect their compliance with treatment and their willingness to adopt health behaviours.

- Good health is a positive concept which can be rated highly in the absence or presence of illness or disease.
- The beliefs of patients and families about CVD may vary from those of health professionals, and will require clarification in order to tailor support.
- Misconceptions can cause emotional distress, guilt, and low self-esteem.
- Misconceptions can stimulate the adoption of passive coping strategies such as avoidance and denial and overdependence on health professionals.

So how can health professionals help people to change?

There are lots of theories that contribute to our understanding of the psychological determinants of health behaviour. See Box 5.2.

Box 5.2 Some empirical models of social cognition

- Health belief model
- Protection motivation theory
- Theory of reasoned action
- Theory of planned behaviour
- Health locus of control
- Social learning theory
- Theory of self-efficacy
- Transtheoretical model

Figure 5.1 outlines a theoretical framework of how these theories together explain behaviour.

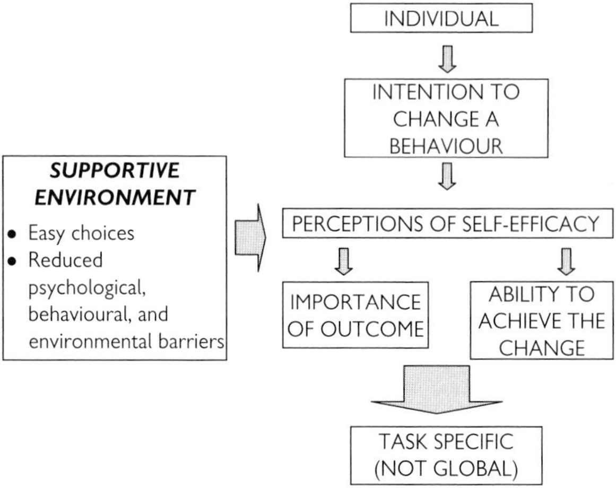

Fig. 5.1 A theoretical framework for behavioural change.

An approach to facilitating behavioural change

The approach described below draws on the motivational interviewing techniques developed by Rollnick and Miller. The principles of motivational interviewing are outlined below.

- A directive, client-centred counselling style for eliciting behaviour change by helping clients explore and resolve ambivalence.
- Aims to increase internal motivation for change rather than impose change.
- Exchange information—assess motivation—brainstorm solutions.

This method has been shown to be superior to traditional advice given for a broad range of behavioural problems and diseases. The effectiveness of this approach improves with increased number and length of encounters, and one-to-one versus group sessions. However, motivational interviewing can be effective even with brief encounters of only 15 minutes.

The specialists from the multidisciplinary team should integrate these counselling techniques into their work with patients and their families, in helping them to stop smoking, to adopt a cardioprotective diet, to become more physically active, and to lose weight.

Establish a rapport

- Use the 'OARS' principles (Fig. 5.2).
- Listen carefully.
- Clarify your understanding by reflecting what patients have said back to them, i.e. repeat, paraphrase, and/or summarize what they have said.

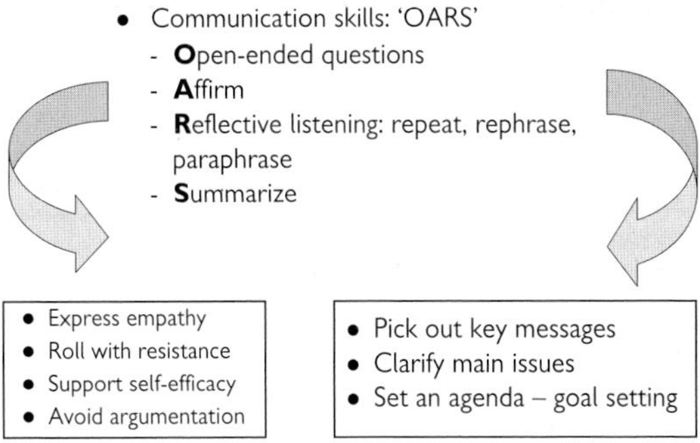

Communication skills: 'OARS'
- Open-ended questions
- Affirm
- Reflective listening: repeat, rephrase, paraphrase
- Summarize
Express empathy
Roll with resistance
Support self-efficacy
Avoid argumentation
Pick out key messages
Clarify main issues
Set an agenda – goal setting

Fig. 5.2 OARS—basic principles.

Set the agenda

- Set an agenda according to the patient's priorities.
- Ask if it is OK to talk about behaviour change.
- Ask what they want to talk about.
- Agree on what is to be covered in the present consultation, and what will be covered in future consultations.
- Include plans for action and follow-up.

Assess motivation and readiness to change

Motivation is a mixture of the importance a person places on a change, the confidence they have to carry out the change and their readiness to change.

- Use scaling questions to assess importance and confidence. Scaling questions (1–10; How important is it for you to change? How confident do you feel? Why so high? What would it take to move you one step higher?) (see Fig. 5.3).
- The ***Stages of change model or transtheoretical model*** (see Fig. 5.4) proposed by Prochaska *et al.*[1] provides one way of assessing readiness to change. The model proposes five stages: pre-contemplation, contemplation, preparation, action, and maintenance.

1 Prochaska, J.O., DiClemente, C.C., and Norcross, J.C. (1992). In search of how people change: applications to addictive behaviour. *American Psychologist*, **47**, 1102–14.

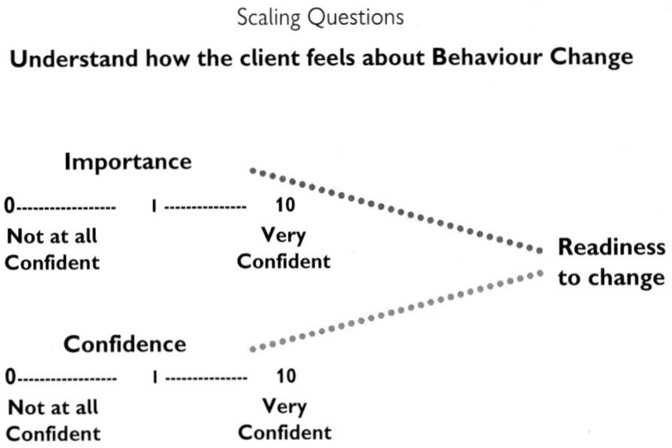

Fig. 5.3 Scaling questions: understand how the client feels about behaviour change.

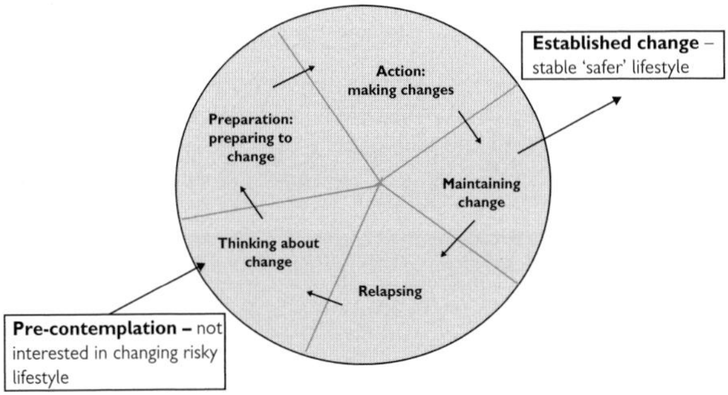

Fig. 5.4 Stages of change model or transtheoretical model.

Exchanging information

The 'elicit–provide–elicit' model is useful for exchanging information with patients:

- ***Elicit***: What do you want to know? What do you know?
- ***Provide***: Clear and neutral information.
- ***Elicit***: What do you make of this?

Selected relevant information can be given to patients to take away if they wish. It is important to remember that you are the expert for the facts and the patient is the expert for what will work for them.

Develop discrepancy

- Increasing awareness in the client of a discrepancy of where he/she is and where he/she wants to be can help to motivate change.
- Affirm key values and an awareness of consequences. The patient, and not the professional, should present the arguments for change.
- Be careful not to provoke negative thoughts and bring to the surface feelings of low self-esteem when using this technique.

Rolling with resistance

- Resistance can be seen in terms of four categories: arguing, interrupting, denying, and ignoring. Work with the patient when he/she is resisting, and avoid arguing with them.
- Emphasize their personal control. Resistance can be a sign to the professional to change strategies.
- Resistance is a sign to the professional that they should respond differently—and not a sign that the patient is 'being difficult'.
- Accept resistance and flow with it, using reflective listening.
- Empathize and show that you understand the patient's dilemma/problem, rather than confront them about their resistance.
- Emphasize personal choice and control over decisions to change.
- Reassess readiness, importance, confidence, and barriers to change.

Exploring options and agreeing on decisions about actions and follow-up

- Elicit from the patient the changes they feel they could make, rather than telling them what to do.
- Help patients to make decisions for themselves.
- Respect the person's values and autonomy—accept that only they can decide to change.
- Allow the patient to resolve his/her uncertainties about change and to set the agenda for behaviour change.
- Support self-confidence, especially in ability to change.
- For each behaviour change, agree on *achievable* goals and strategies (see Fig. 5.5).
- Agree on plans to follow up by telephone, consultation, or referral.

Goal setting

- **S**pecific
- **M**easurable
- **A**chievable
- **R**eliable
- **T**imely

A contract is agreed between yourself and the patient

↓

'Ownership' of goals

Signs it is working

- Patient is doing most of the talking
- Patient is actively talking about change
- Patient is working hard and realizing things for first time
- Sense of partnership between patient and professional

Things to avoid

- Confrontation, labelling, blaming
- Direct persuasion
- Commanding approach/threatening language (giving advice, moralizing, shaming)
- Simple solutions
- Dangerous assumptions (patients are either motivated or not, expert trap)

Respect the patient's decision

Fig. 5.5 Setting achievable goals.

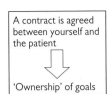

Overcoming negative thought processes

Important behavioural changes will be more effectively achieved in the absence of anxiety, distress, and negative thought processes, which may have been provoked by any of the following:

- Misconceptions about the disease process
- Depression
- Erroneous health beliefs.

These dysfunctional thoughts may be identified by the professional through discussions with the patient and his or her partner, and also from the questionnaires that are completed as part of the multidisciplinary assessment regarding anxiety, depression, mood, and perceptions about illness and risk (see Chapter 4).

Cognitive behavioural therapy (CBT) provides a proven effective model to manage negative thought processes. CBT helps by:

- Breaking problems down into smaller parts, making it easier to see how each part is connected and how they affect an individual.
- Uncovering the underlying thoughts, emotions, physical feelings, and actions.
- Breaking the cycle of negative feelings and behaviour.

CBT is effective in a wide range of conditions, particularly anxiety, depression, and post-traumatic stress disorder, and has been used successfully with angina patients.

Key references

Department of Health (2001). *Treatment choice in psychological therapies and counselling – an evidence based clinical practice guideline.* London: Department of Health.

Kaptein, A. and Weinman, J. (eds). (2004). *Health psychology*, (1st edn). Oxford: Blackwell Publishing.

Rollnick, S., Mason, P., and Butler, C. (1999). *Health behavior change. A guide for practitioners*, (1st edn). Edinburgh: Churchill Livingstone.

Rubak, S., Sandboek, A., Lauritzen, T., and Christensen, B. (2005). Motivational interviewing. A systematic review and meta-analysis. *British Journal of General Practice*, **55**, 305–12.

Tones, K. and Green, J. (2004). *Health promotion. Planning and strategies*, (1st edn). London: Sage Publications.

Chapter 6
Smoking cessation

Two strategies to help people to stop smoking:

- Offer brief advice
- Provide behavioural support plus drug therapy
  BOTH ARE HIGHLY COST EFFECTIVE AND SAVE LIVES

How does brief advice help?

- Opportunistic advice raises the sense of urgency
- Increases the probability of a future quit attempt
- Offers a hope of success with proven effective therapies
- Attempts to get committment
- May increase the effectiveness of a future quit attempt

The challenge of helping high-risk patients to stop smoking

Patients with symptomatic atherosclerotic disease, those at high risk of developing disease, and their partners are from an older age group (usually over 50 years). The smokers among them will:

- have been smoking for many years and will be less likely to want to stop or be lacking in confidence to achieve it
- be more physically dependent on nicotine
- will need both counselling and pharmacological support to succeed.

For the most part, they will come from a lower socio-economic group where the prevalence of atherosclerotic disease and cardiovascular risk factors is higher.

How to structure advice

Box 6.1 The five A's

- ASK about tobacco use at every visit
- ADVISE tobacco users to quit
- ASSESS readiness to quit
- ASSIST tobacco users with a quit plan
- ARRANGE follow-up visits

Box 6.2 The 30 second Approach- ABC

• ASK-	ask and record smoking status
• BRIEF ADVICE-	'stopping smoking is the best thing you can do for your health'
• CONFIDENCE	-Encourage and build self confidence -Tell smokers about effective therapies to aid quitting -Refer to help www.nhs.uk/smokefree

Box 6.3 Preparing to Stop Now

- Set the quit date, preferably within 2 weeks.
- Assess the availability of social support, e.g. from family.
- Ask about what worked in past quit attempts and the perceived cause of lapses.
- Discuss concerns, e.g. weight gain.
- Make a contingency plan to prevent relapse.
- Discuss using pharmacological support such as nicotine replacement therapy (NRT), bupropion, or varenicline.
- Refer to resources such as national helpline and written materials.
- Arrange a follow-up date, either face to face or by telephone.

Some facts about weight gain and smoking cessation

- The net effect of quitting smoking is an average of 7kg weight gain which is permanent
- The higher the BMI at the time of quitting the greater the weight gain
- The benefits of stopping smoking outweigh the disadvantages of weight gain
- Cognitive behaviour therapy may reduce weight gain during a quit attempt.

Advise people trying to quit to eat healthy snacks and to be physically active

Preventing relapse

Smoking is an addiction and a chronic relapsing condition. A relapse during a quit attempt should not be seen as a failure but as a learning experience and a first step towards success. Only 20% of smokers manage to permanently stop smoking on their first attempt.

Considerations in helping patients to develop a contingency plan to avoid relapse

- Change routines-old cues to smoking are the most important trigger.
- Negative mood is the second most important trigger
- Alcohol may weaken resolve during a quit attempt
- Lapses are more likely to happen in the evening
- Stick to 'not a puff' advice-90% of lapses lead to a full relapse
- Practice assertiveness in dealing with social pressure.
- Prepare for anxiety, e.g. relaxation techniques, positive self-talk.
- Identify positive social support networks.
- Extended use of pharmatherapies like NRT may be useful in preventing relapse.

Depression

- Nicotine may have antidepressant effects. Its withdrawal may precipitate depressive symptoms.
- Always treat depression before embarking on smoking cessation.
- Proceed with caution in people susceptible to depression (e.g. with a history).

Always follow up a patient who has set a quit date

Tobacco treatments

Using treatments and getting individual or group counselling support is associated with more successful quit attempts than going 'cold turkey'.

- NRT (patches, gum, etc.)
- Nicotine receptor partial agonists (varenicline)
- Antidepressants (bupropion)

Box 6.4 Prescribing NRT

- Prescribe a nicotine patch to deliver a background dose of nicotine in order to reduce withdrawal symptoms.
- In combination, prescribe nicotine nasal spray, inhalator, or gum to deliver nicotine boosts during the course of the day.
- NRT can be used for prolonged periods of up to 9 months in people who are heavily dependent.
- Monitor tolerance of the product being used and be sure to use the correct dose—do not be tempted to underdose.

How to dose NRT

- Assess physical dependence—in particular, time to first cigarette in the morning and number smoked per day (see the Fagerström Test for Nicotine Dependence, Table 4.4).
- If very physically dependent and/or smoking more than twenty cigarettes per day, consider starting with the highest dose (21 mg) 24-hour patch for at least 4 weeks and then titrate to lower doses as dependence is reduced.
- 16-hour patches are also available for people who suffer from insomnia and vivid dreams—this patch is not worn overnight.
- The nasal spray is very useful in those who are heavily physically dependent (smoking more than 20 per day). The dose ranges from 8 to 64 sprays per day.
- The inhalator is useful in people who are very behaviour dependent. The dose ranges from 6 to 16 cartridges per day.
- The gum is useful in moderately behaviour-dependent smokers and mimics the peaks and troughs of smoking. It can also be useful to prevent overeating during an attempt to quit. Up to 24 pieces of either the 2 mg or 4 mg gum can be used per day.

NRT is safe to use with patients who have coronary heart disease

Heavily dependent smokers who want to quit

- Assess physical dependence on nicotine using the FTND (see Table 4.4).
- Tobacco treatment therapies should be an essential part of helping heavily dependent smokers to quit.
- An abrupt attempt to quit may be unrealistic.
- ASH (www.ash.co.uk) have proposed a protocol for reducing cigarette consumption using NRT in the run-up to a quit attempt.
- Evidence is emerging about pre-treatment with NRT prior to a quit attempt to increase success.

Box 6.5 ASH: Nicotine Assisted Reduction to Stop (licensing arrangements for NRT in the UK allow the use of this protocol)

0–6 weeks	Cut down to 50% of initial consumption
6 weeks to 9 months	Continue to cut down and aim to stop completely by 6 months
6–9 months	Stop smoking completely and continue to use NRT
Within 12 months	Stop using NRT by 12 months

ASH recommends:

- Prescriptions be issued 2 weeks at a time.
- No repeat prescriptions should be issued during the cut-down period unless daily reduction is reported.
- Reduction should be validated with breath CO readings.
- Once an individual decides to quit completely, calculate the NRT dose on the basis of initial tobacco consumption.

Box 6.6 Prescribing nicotine receptor partial agonists (varenicline)

- Set the quit date for between 1 and 2 weeks after the individual starts to take varenicline.
- Gradually increase the dose over this period from 0.5 mg daily to 1 mg twice daily—this helps to prevent nausea.
- Usual length of therapy is 12 weeks (this can be repeated to help sustain a quit attempt in the long term).

Box 6.7 Prescribing bupropion

- Set the quit date for between 1 and 2 weeks after the individual starts to take bupropion.
- Increase the dose from 150 mg every morning for 6 days to 150 mg twice daily.
- The treatment should be continued for between 7 and 9 weeks.

Smoking cessation guidelines

UK: National Institute for Clinical Excellence (NICE) www.nice.org.uk
-Brief Interventions March 2006 PH1001
-Smoking cessation services in primary case, pharmacies, local authorities and workplaces February 2008 PH1010
-Vatenicline for smoking cessation July 2007 TA123

USA: www.ahrq.gov

Key references and websites

Britton, J., Bates, C., Channer, K., *et al.* (2000). *Nicotine addiction in Britain*. Tobacco Advisory Group of the Royal College of Physicians, UK.

Hubbard, R., Lewis, S., Smith, C., *et al.* (2005). Use of nicotine replacement therapy and the risk of acute myocardial infarction, stroke and death. *Tobacco Control*, **14**, 416–21.

Wu, P., Wilson, K., Dimoulas, P., *et al.* (2005). Effectiveness of smoking cessation therapies: a systematic review and meta-analysis. *BMC Public Health*, 6 December, 300.

www.rjwest.co.uk

West, R. (2008). Smoking tool kit study: www.smokinginengland.inf

Chapter 7

Principles of dietary intervention

The aim of dietary intervention is to help families make appropriate changes to their diet to bring it in line with a cardioprotective diet.

Principles of dietary intervention[1]

Information from assessment

Using the data collected in the dietary assessment, it will be possible to identify the family's

- pattern of eating and drinking
- amount of eating and drinking
- nutrient excess or deficiency
- barriers to change
- motivation level and stage of change
- knowledge and understanding level
- support needs

Developing a successful relationship with the patient and partner

Discussing dietary habits and weight issues can be a sensitive issue. Some of the following techniques and attitudes may be helpful to develop a successful partnership with families to help them change:

- Reflective listening
- Empathy
- Being sympathetic and sensitive to personal issues
- Being realistic
- Being personable

Types of interventions

Dietary advice can be provided to families using different strategies:

- Group sessions
- Individual consultations
- Videos
- Cooking lessons
- Written literature

Negotiating goals and developing a change plan

Agreeing appropriate behavioural changes/goals is key to achieving positive outcomes.

- Patients/families must play an active role in defining realistic changes.
- Unrealistic goals can lead to failure or reduce compliance.
- It is essential to take on board other lifestyle factors.
- Not too many goals should be set at one time.
- Define a time to review progress and reward scheme (non-food based).
- Identify triggers that may cause relapse and make a contingency plan.
- Discuss and identify ways families can self-monitor themselves.

(See Chapter 5 for more details.)

Box 7.1 Ideally goals should fulfil the SMART criteria

Specific: grilling the fish rather than frying it will help to reduce fat intake
Measurable: try to have one piece of fruit and one vegetable each day
Achievable and realistic: try to reduce biscuits to two with each coffee rather than four
Relevant to goal of treatment: if the aim of the treatment is to reduce blood pressure, goals should help the patient concentrate on reducing salt and increasing potassium from fruit and vegetables
Time specific: keep a food diary for 3 days

Frequency of intervention

An agreed follow-up, monitoring, and support plan is essential for positive outcome. Developing a plan for each family on how each of these will be provided will aid a secure and productive relationship.

Need for family involvement

The need for family involvement is particularly important for the diet. Patients trying to change their diet in isolation at home are going to find it more difficult to make changes alone than with the support of the family (see Chapter 1, Why families too?).

1 Thomas, B., Bishop, Y. (2007). Manual or dietetic practice 4th ed. *Blackwell*

What is a cardioprotective diet?

The Mediterranean dietary pattern is associated with a decreased risk of CVD. It has a high unsaturated to saturated fat ratio; high intake of legumes, nuts, seeds, grains, fruit, vegetables, potatoes, and fish, and a low intake of meat and meat products; fresh rather than processed foods are consumed.

The cardioprotective diet is thought to exert its effects on CVD by having a positive effect on different risk factors. These include blood pressure, lipid profile, insulin resistance, platelet aggregation, clotting factors, arrhythmias, homocysteine levels, and inflammation.

Table 7.1 The recommendations for a cardioprotective diet

	General population	Those at high CVD multi-factorial risk or with CVD
Balanced diet	A wide variety of food should be eaten	A wide variety of food should be eaten
Fat	Replace saturated with unsaturated fat (monounsaturated and polyunsaturated) where possible. Total daily energy from fat <30%	Replace saturated with unsaturated fat (monounsaturated and polyunsaturated) where possible Total daily energy from fat <30%
Fish	2+ portions of fish weekly, one of which should be oily	2+ portions of fish weekly, one of which should be oily (Post MI, oily fish should be consumed 2-4 portions/week (1 portion=140g). If not possible, replace with a supplement (1 g eicosapentaenoic acid (EPA)/docosahexaenoic acid (DHA)/day)
Fruit and vegetables	At least 5 portions a day	At least 5 portions a day
Soluble fibre	Regular intake of beans, pulses, legumes, rice, pasta	Regular intake of beans, pulses, legumes, rice, pasta
Salt	Limited intake (<6 g/day; reduction in processed foods)	Limited intake (<6 g/day; reduction in processed foods)
Alcohol	Moderate intake: Women <14 units/week or <2-3 units/day with 2 alcohol free days/week Men <21 units/week or <3-4 units/day with 2 alcohol free days per week	Moderate intake: Women <14 units/week or <2-3 units/day with 2 alcohol free days/week Men <21 units/week or <3-4 units/day with 2 alcohol free days per week
Energy intake	Maintenance of energy balance to prevent weight gain	Maintenance of energy balance to prevent weight gain

Box 7.2 Examples of possible options for a cardioprotective diet

Breakfast

- Fresh fruit or fruit juice
- Porridge/wholegrain cereal with low-fat milk
- Wholegrain bread, thinly spread with unsaturated fat spread
- For the occasional cooked breakfast, try: boiled or poached egg, grilled lean bacon, baked or grilled tomatoes, or baked beans on wholegrain toast
- Tea, coffee, sugar-free drink

Snack meal

- Wholegrain sandwich with low-fat filling, e.g. cottage cheese, chicken, tuna, salmon, ham and salad
- Baked beans/sardines/poached egg on toast with salad
- Home-made vegetable and bean soup
- Jacket potato and beans, tuna, or cottage cheese

Mid morning/afternoon

- Tea, coffee, sugar-free drink
- Fruit, low-fat yoghurt or high-fibre snack

Main meal

- Small serving of lean meat/fish/egg or large serving of beans or lentils
- Large serving of vegetables or salad (aim for half the plate)
- Potatoes, wholegrain bread, rice, pasta, chapatti, yam, or plantain
- *For dessert*: fruit, low-fat yoghurt, low-fat and low-sugar puddings

Drinks

- Water, tea, coffee (in moderation), sugar-free drinks, and small quantities of fruit juice

Fats

A cardioprotective diet is quite high in fat but the ratio of saturated to unsaturated is what appears to help prevent cardiovascular disease. It is often misconceived that a cardioprotective diet is low in fat.

Fat is an essential part of the diet, required for:

- Energy for cells through oxidation
- Providing essential fatty acids
- Carrier for fat-soluble vitamins (A, D, E, and K) and antioxidants
- Acting as a protective layer around organs
- Essential structural, storage, and metabolic functions
- Improving food flavour and palatability
- Growth and development.

Fats are usually grouped into three main types depending on their structure:

Type of fat	Recommended intake	Structure
Saturated fatty acids (SFA)	≤10% total energy	Carbon atoms only linked by single bonds; solid at room temperature
Monounsaturated fatty acids (MUFA)	≥13% total energy	Contain one double bond; liquid at room temperature
Polyunsaturated fatty acids (PUFA)	≥6% total energy	Contain two or more double bonds; liquid at room temperature. Divided into two types, omega-3 and omega-6, which have different metabolic effects

Trans fatty acids are also found, these have a similar metabolic effect as saturated fats and are formed artificially during hydrogenation of unsaturated oils:

Trans fatty acids (TFA)	≤2% total energy	Unsaturated fats come in either the *cis*- (hydrogen on the same side) or *trans*- (hydrogen on opposite sides) form

To identify the fat content on food labels the following can be used as a guide:[2]

	per 100 g		
	Low	Moderate	High
Total fat	<3 g	2–20 g	>20 g
Saturated fat	<1.5 g	1.5-5 g	>5 g

Table 7.2 Fats: sources and implications for CVD

Type of fat	Where it is found	Effect on CVD risk factors
SFA	Animal products: meat fat, cheese, cream, butter, dripping, pastry, ghee Plant products: coconut, palm oil	Increase LDL Increase total cholesterol Enhances atherosclerosis development
MUFA	Olive oil Rapeseed oil Groundnut oil Nuts and seeds Avocado	Reduces total and LDL cholesterol when substituting for saturated fat No effect on HDL Less risk of lipid peroxidation than polyunsaturated fat
omega-3 PUFA	Oils: walnut, soybean, flaxseed Oily fish: mackerel, salmon, sardines, trout, pilchards, herrings Enriched products: eggs, milk, yogurt	Minimal effect on blood cholesterol Very high doses reduce triglycerides Antithrombotic, anti-arrhythmic, and anti-inflammatory effect
omega-6 PUFA	Oils: sunflower, safflower, corn, groundnut, and soya	Reduces LDL and total cholesterol, but very high doses may reduce HDL, enhance lipid peroxidation, and free-radical production
Trans fatty acids	Dairy products, cakes, biscuits, processed foods, deep-fried fat foods	Increase LDL, increase total cholesterol Enhances atherosclerosis development

Practical tips to reduce saturated fat intake

- Avoid obvious high sources of SFA (visible fat, creamy sauces, pastry, cakes, biscuits).
- Be vigilant about removing fat in the cooking process.
- Reduce the amount of fat added to cooking by measuring it out.
- Limit the intake of cheese and cheese sauces.
- Try not to fry with butter, ghee, or palm oil. Try to steam, boil, microwave, or bake instead.
- Choose leaner meats and leaner cuts of meat where possible.
- Choose lower-fat options.
- Change the proportions on your plate so you have more vegetables than protein or carbohydrate.

2 http://www.food.gov.uk/multimedia/pdfs/publication/whichcard0908.pdf

Fish and oily fish

Fish is a great source of protein, vitamins, and minerals. It is usually classed as either white or oily fish, both can be part of a cardioprotective diet.

- ***White fish***: e.g. cod, haddock, plaice, skate, halibut, john dory, sole, coley, whiting, sea bass, sea bream.
- ***Oily fish***: e.g. mackerel, salmon, sardines, pilchards, trout, herrings, trout, tuna, anchovies, swordfish.

When preparing fish, remember to use methods that are healthy—poaching, microwaving, or grilling, rather than frying in batter or breadcrumbs.

Oily fish and heart disease

The omega-3 fatty acids (EPA and DHA) in oily fish have been shown to be protective against heart disease by:

- Reducing mortality after myocardial infarction
- Reducing arrythmias
- Modulating blood platelet activity and tendency to thrombosis
- High doses (supplementation of 3 g/day) reduce triglycerides.

Recommended intake

- After myocardial infarction:
  - 2–4 large servings of high omega-3 oily fish (Fig. 7.1) weekly
  - OR 1 g (EPA and DHA) omega-3 supplement per day
- All other patient groups:
  - 1 serving of oily fish and a minimum of one white fish per week

Serving size

- This depends on the type of fish. A rough serving size is 100–150 g (4–6 oz) of fresh, frozen, or smoked fish or one small, half a medium or one-third of a large tin of canned fish.
- If possible, buy local or fish from environmentally friendly sources.
- Limit smoked fish to no more than once a week.

Vegetarian sources of omega-3 PUFA

Alpha-linolenic acid can be converted into the protective EPA and DHA. Unfortunately this is a very ineffective process and therefore it is extremely difficult to obtain adequate amounts. Omega-3 contents can vary greatly, so check the label.

Vegetarian sources high in omega-3 PUFA include:

- Rapeseed, canola, walnut, soya, flaxseed, linseed oils
- Nuts: walnuts, pecans, almonds, peanuts
- Soybean and tofu
- Dark-green leafy vegetables, sweet potato, and wholegrains
- Omega-3 enriched foods—eggs, milk, yoghurt.

OMEGA - 3 FATS FOUND IN FISH – per average serving
High sources of omega-3 are above the dotted line

Mackerel – fresh or frozen	**Very High Source**
Kippers – fresh, frozen or canned	
Pilchards – canned in tomato sauce	↑
Tuna or trout – fresh or frozen	
Sprats or salmon – fresh or frozen	
Mackerel – smoked or canned	
Sardines – fresh or canned	
Herring – pickled, fresh or frozen	
Sild or skippers – canned	
Salmon – canned in brine or in pasta dishes or smoked salmon	
Crab– fresh	
Herring – cann	
Trout – smokeded	
Swordfish (only eat swordfish, shark and marln once a week)	
Salmon fish cakes or potato-toppped pies	
Salmon Fish Paté	
... ...	... ...
Tuna– canned in oil	
Crab – canned in brine	
Eel – fresh or jellied	
Fish paste –Crab, Salmon, Sardine	
Cod or haddock – fresh or frozen	
Fish cakes or fish fingers (white)	
Tuna– canned in brine or water	
	Low Source

Fig. 7.1 Fish containing omega-3 fatty acids. Reproduced with kind permission from Rachel Vine and UKHHDSG of the British Dietetic Association.

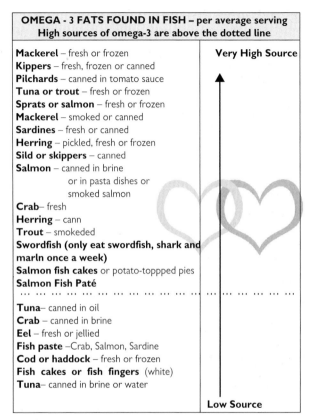

Fruit and vegetables

Fruit and vegetables are an essential part of the cardioprotective diet. A variety of fruit and vegetable should be included in the diet.

They are beneficial for the prevention of many chronic diseases, including heart disease, as they are:

- High in soluble fibre and therefore have a low glycaemic index
- High in antioxidants
- High in folic acid
- Low in fat and calories.

How does this reduce risk?

- Reduces cholesterol levels by reducing fat absorption.
- Protects against formation of oxidized low-density lipoprotein.
- Protects against free radicals.
- Reduces homocysteine levels.
- Reduces blood pressure.
- Helps with weight management.
- Improves gut transit time.
- Improves glycaemic control, especially in diabetics.

Recommended intake

- Minimum of five portions (Box 7.3) each day.
- This can be a combination of fruit and vegetables.
- Try to have a variety of colours to get different vitamins and minerals.
- Fresh, frozen, or tinned in natural juices are OK.
- Fruit juice/smoothies only count as one portion.
- Potatoes do not count.

Are there any fruits and vegetables that should be avoided?

The only fruit to avoid is grapefruit (and grapefruit juice) if the patient is taking certain statins—check the tablet information leaflet.

Vitamin supplements

An adequate amount of vitamins and minerals is achievable if a varied balanced meal is consumed.

Box 7.3 Portion sizes of fruit and vegetables: what is a portion?

Fruit:

Apricot, dried	3 whole
Apricot, fresh	3 apricots
Banana, fresh	1 medium banana
Blueberries	2 handfuls (4 heaped tbsp)
Clementines	2 clementines
Fruit juice	1 × 150 ml glass
Fruit salad, canned	3 heaped tablespoons
Fruit smoothie	1 × 150ml glass
Grapes	1 handful
Mango	2 slices (2-inch slice)
Melon	1 slice (2-inch slice)
Mixed fruit, dried	1 heaped tablespoon
Nectarine/peach	1 nectarine
Orange	1 orange
Pear, canned	2 halves or 7 slices
Pineapple, canned	2 rings or 12 chunks
Plum	2 medium plums
Prune, canned	6 prunes
Strawberry, fresh	7 strawberries
Sultanas	1 heaped tablespoon

Vegetables:

Asparagus, fresh	5 spears
Aubergine	1/3rd aubergine
Beans, broad/butter/kidney cooked	3 heaped tablespoons
Beans, French/runner cooked	4 heaped tablespoons
Beansprouts, fresh	2 handfuls
Beetroot, bottled	3 'baby' whole, or 7 slices
Broccoli	2 spears
Brussel sprouts	8 Brussel sprouts
Carrots, fresh/canned slices	3 heaped tablespoons
Cauliflower	8 florets
Celery	3 sticks
Leeks	1 leek (white portion only)
Lentils	3 tablespoons
Lettuce (mixed leaves)	1 cereal bowl
Mixed vegetables, frozen	3 tablespoons
Onion, fresh	1 medium onion
Parsnips	1 large
Peas, canned/fresh/frozen	3 heaped tablespoons
Spinach, cooked	2 heaped tablespoons
Spring greens, cooked	4 heaped tablespoons
Tomato, fresh	1 medium, or 7 cherry

Carbohydrate and fibre

Carbohydrates are the main source of energy and are derived from plant foods. Carbohydrates are often split into two groups but this divide is not clear-cut.

- Digestible carbohydrate (postprandial rise in blood glucose) is broken down to produce glucose which is essential for brain and body tissue function.
- Non-digestible carbohydrates (no postprandial rise in blood glucose) have important gastrointestinal function. It is thought that these may be absorbed in the colon following fermentation.

Glycaemic index (GI)[3]

The glycaemic index describes the effect that different carbohydrates have on glucose levels. Low GI carbohydrates (Table 7.3) produce only small fluctuations in our blood glucose and insulin levels. This is important for long-term health and reducing risk of heart disease and diabetes.

Benefits of a low-GI diet

- Weight management
- Increases insulin sensitivity
- Improves diabetes control
- Reduces the risk of heart disease
- Improves lipid profiles
- Helps manage the symptoms of polycystic ovarian syndrome (PCOS)
- Reduces hunger and keeps you fuller for longer
- Prolongs physical endurance

Table 7.3 GI of different food groups

	Low GI	Medium GI	High GI
Rice	Basmati	Brown/white	
Bread	Wholegrain, granary	Pitta, muffin, croissant	Baguette, bagel, wholemeal
Cereals	Oat-based (e.g. porridge, muesli), bran rich	Cereal bars	Wheat- or maize-based (e.g. cornflakes, Weetabix)
Potatoes	New potatoes in skin	Boiled old potatoes, chips	Mashed, instant, jacket potatoes
Fruit	Most fruits	Dried fruit, banana, pineapple	Fruit juice, watermelon, lychees
Vegetables	All green and salad vegetables, carrots, yam	Sweet potato, sweetcorn, beetroot	Pumpkin, parsnips
Dairy Foods	Plain yoghurt, milk		Flavoured yoghurt
Sugar	Fructose	Sucrose, honey	Glucose, lucozade

The GI of a food will also vary depending on how it is cooked, processed, prepared (ingredients), or its ripeness. It is also rare for foods to be eaten in isolation, therefore it is important to think of the glycaemic load—this is the effect on postprandial glucose that the whole meal will have, rather than the individual foods, e.g. combining a high-GI food with a low-GI foods will lead to a medium-GI load (jacket potato and baked beans, for example).

Dietary fibre

This is described as the substance that is not digested by enzymes but which may undergo fermentation on reaching the colon. They are divided into different types:

Type	Role	Sources
Soluble fibre	Reduces postprandial lipid and glucose absorption	Pulses, beans, oats, fruit, and vegetables
Insoluble fibre	Increases stool weight and transit time	Bran, potato skins, seeds, wholemeal products, nuts
Resistant starch	Fermentation produces short-chain fatty acids	Modified starch, potato, green banana, rice, bread
Prebiotics, fructo-oligosaccharides, fructans	Equilibrate gut flora, laxation, fermentation produces short-chain fatty acids	Functional foods—added to products—leeks, banana, onion
Indigestible animal products	Cholesterol lowering	Seafood shells
Phytates	Reduce absorption of calcium, zinc, and iron. Thought to protect against cancer due to the reduced absorption of iron, which reduces cell growth	Legumes, grains, soybean

Ways to increase fibre intake

- Choose wholegrain products.
- Use wholemeal flour or use half white, half brown.
- Eat the skins on fruit and vegetables.
- Add fruit, nuts, and seeds to cereals and salads.
- Do not mash or blend fruit and vegetables.

Remember to increase fluid intake when increasing fibre intake

3 Ludwig, D. (2002). The glycaemic index physicological mechanisms relating to obesity, diabetes and cardiovascular disease. *JAMA* vol 287 pp.2414-23.

Protein

Proteins are comprised of amino acids. They are the building blocks of the body, managing metabolism and organ function.

There are three types of amino acids:

- Essential—not synthesized by the body so must be in diet.
- Non-essential—readily synthesized by body.
- Conditionally essential—can be synthesized but may be needed from the diet under certain circumstances.

Protein requirements

- Healthy adult: 0.75–0.83 g protein/kg ideal body weight/day.
- The average intake in the UK is usual well above this level.
- During pregnancy or lactation requirements increase.

Protein sources

Protein is obtained from both animal and plant sources:

- Animal: meat, fish, poultry, eggs
- Plant: pulses, legumes, soya, nuts, beans.

The majority of people in the UK and Europe get most of their protein from animal sources. These sources are often associated with excessive saturated fat and therefore can be detrimental to prevention of CVD.

Ways to reduce saturated fat from protein sources

- Remove all visible fat prior to cooking (including chicken skin).
- Choose lean cuts of meat.
- Choose low-fat dairy options.
- Try not to fry; poach, grill, or bake instead.

Soya protein

Including soya protein in the diet may beneficial for reducing CVD risk. Benefits of replacing lean meat with soya protein:

- Decreases total cholesterol, LDL, and triglycerides without altering HDL concentrations.
- Replacement of meat with soya protein will decrease saturated fat intake and increase the PUFA:SFA ratio, hence a having a beneficial effect on plasma lipoprotein levels.
- May also be protective against LDL oxidation susceptibility.

Observations from the Anderson trial[4] suggest that the daily consumption of 31–47 g of soya protein can significantly decrease serum cholesterol and LDL cholesterol concentration (ingestion of 25 or 50 g of soya protein/day was estimated to decrease serum cholesterol concentration by 0.23 mmol/l and 0.45 mmol/l, respectively).

4 Anderson, J.W., Johnstone, B.M., and Cook-Newell, M.E. (1995). Meta-analysis of the effects of soy protein intake on serum lipids. *New England Journal of Medicine*, **333**(5), 276–82.

Persons with hypercholesterolaemia can achieve an intake of more than 30 g of soya protein/day by consuming 2–3 servings of soya products daily.

8 oz (226 g) soya milk	≡ 4–10 g protein
4 oz (113 g) tofu	≡ 8–13 g protein
1 oz (28 g) soya flour	≡ 10–13 g protein
4 oz (113 g) textured protein	≡ 11 g protein
3 oz (90 g) meat analogue	≡ 18 g protein

Therefore 2 cups of soya milk and 1 portion of meat replacement ≡ 30 g soya protein and has a significant effect.

Alcohol

Recommended safe intake of alcohol for people at risk of CVD:

see Table 7.1, p. 126.

Alcohol is not an essential nutrient. The relationship between alcohol and total mortality has a U or J shape. Non-drinkers have a slightly higher risk than moderate drinkers. This does not mean that non-drinkers should start drinking.

Possible benefits of alcohol

- Increases HDL.
- Inhibition of platelet aggregation.

Observational studies suggest that wine does not appear to be any more beneficial than any other type of alcohol.[5]

Possible problems with high alcohol intake (>3 units/day for women; >4 units/day for men)

- Can be additive.
- High in calories (7 kcal/g).
- Detrimental to the liver.
- Raises blood pressure.
- Raises triglycerides.
- Results in poor blood sugar control in diabetics.
- Binge drinking can particularly affect cardiac muscle.

Optimal consumption is lower for women than for men because of enzymatic differences in alcohol metabolism in women.

Mixer drinks should be sugar free. Consumption of low-carbohydrate beers and 'low-alcohol' drinks are not preferable because of their higher sugar and energy content.

Note

Most people underestimate their alcohol intake. It has also been observed that those who drink more often have a higher intake of salt which, in turn, could affect their blood pressure. Therefore, each case should be considered individually.

Table 7.4 Alcohol content in different drinks

Drink	Alcohol by volume (ABV)	Measure	No. of units (g)
Beers, lagers and cider	3–5%	250 ml (1/2 pt)	0.75–1.25 (7.5–12.5)
		500 ml (1 pt)	1.5–2.5 (15–25)
	6–8%	250 ml (1/2 pt)	1.5–2.0 (15–20)
		500 ml (1 pt)	3.0–4.0 (30–40)
Wine	9–11%	Small glass (125 ml)	1.0–1.4 (10–14)
		Medium glass (175 ml)	1.6–2.0 (16–20)
		Large glass (250 ml)	2.25–2.75(22.5–27.5)
		1 bottle	6.75–8.25(67.5–82.5)
	12–14%	Small glass (125 ml)	1.5–1.75(15–17.5)
		Medium glass (175 ml)	2.1–2.45 (21–24.5)
		Large glass (250 ml)	3.0–3.5 (30–35)
		1 bottle	9.0–10.5 (90–105)
Fortified wine e.g. sherry/port	16%	50 ml glass	0.8 (8.0)
Spirits e.g. vodka/gin	40%	25 ml	1.0 (10)

Suggested ways for patients/families to reduce their alcohol intake

- Drink half pints rather than pints.
- Put your drink down in between sips.
- Sip rather than gulp.
- Be aware of alcohol content in drinks.
- Measure drinks out at home.
- Have soft drinks on the table.
- Move the glass to your non-drinking-hand side.
- Buy smaller glasses for at home.

5 Rimm, E.B., Klatsky, A., Grobbee, D., and Stampfer, M.J. (1996). Review of moderate alcohol consumption and reduced risk of coronary heart disease: is the effect due to beer, wine, or spirits? *British Medical Journal*, **312**(7033), 731–6.

Salt (sodium chloride)

Sodium is an essential nutrient, whose balance in the body is maintained by effective homeostatic mechanisms. It is essential for regulation of fluid balance, blood pressure, and transmembrane gradients. Chloride is also important for fluid balance, gastric, and intestinal secretions. Most intake is from common salt and is eaten is excess of requirements.

Recommended intake

- <6 g/day
- In the UK and Europe the average intake is approx 9 g/day; 75% of this is estimated to come from processed foods.

Effect of a high salt intake

Increases blood pressure and consequently CVD risk.

Benefits of lowering salt intake

- Reduces blood pressure and CVD risk.
- A salt reduction of 3 g/day could lead to a 3.5 mmHg reduction in systolic blood pressure.

Practical advice for lowering salt intake

- Discourage use of salt at the table or in cooking.
- Discourage consumption of foods with a high salt content.
- Encourage the use of alternative ingredients to flavour foods:
    - herbs, spices, lemon juice, garlic, pepper, vinegar, and chilli.
- Do not recommend salt substitutes (e.g. LoSalt).

Box 7.4 Food sources high in salt

- Ready-made meals
- Bread, cereals
- Cheese
- Tinned or packet soups and sauces
- Salted snacks—crisps, nuts
- Sausages, pies, paté
- Smoked meat with added salt
- Stock cubes, meat and vegetable extracts, soy sauce, and marmite

Stanol and sterol esters

Definition

'Functional foods' are foods or dietary components that may provide a health benefit beyond basic nutrition. Examples can include fruits and vegetables, whole grains, fortified or enhanced foods and beverages, and some dietary supplements. Biologically active components in functional foods may impart health benefits or desirable physiological effects. Functional attributes of many traditional foods are being discovered, while new food products are being developed with beneficial components.

Stanol and sterol esters

These are natural products found in many plant products (fruit, vegetables, seeds, nuts, legumes)in small quantities.

- They decrease the absorption of both endogenous and exogenous cholesterol from the intestine. The unabsorbed cholesterol is excreted in the faeces and hence leads to a reduction in total and LDL cholesterol.
- 1.6–2 g/day stanol/sterol esters, is seen as the optimum intake.
- The average cholesterol reduction is about 10%, but individual responses are variable.
- The ability of a stanol or sterol ester to decrease cholesterol does not appear to be significantly different.
- The recommended intake should be eaten each day.
- They are expensive and therefore patients should be made aware of this.
- They can be taken in addition to statins as their cholesterol-lowering mechanism is different. This is not the case for ezitimibe.

1 portion =	1 yoghurt 12 g (2.5 level tsp) of spread 20 g (4 level tsp) of light cream cheese 250 ml milk
OR	1 yoghurt drink/day (70 g or 100 g, depending on make)

Possible problems

They may reduce the absorption of some fat-soluble vitamins, particularly β-carotene. Eating increased amounts of fruit and vegetables could counter the decrease in absorption of the fat-soluble vitamins.

Dietary cholesterol

Recommended intake of dietary cholesterol is less than 300 mg/day

Cholesterol is a wax-like substance that is essential to life as it is the primary component of animal cell membranes and a substrate for the synthesis of bile acids, steroid hormones, and vitamin D.

The influence of dietary cholesterol on blood cholesterol is relatively small because most circulating cholesterol is of endogenous origin. Significant effects are only seen when intake is extremely high, either from foods high in dietary cholesterol or from very high consumption of animal products. There appears to be a tremendous heterogeneity among subjects and individual susceptibilities in response to a low-cholesterol diet.

The evidence that dietary cholesterol, and high-cholesterol foods such as eggs and liver, contribute to CVD risk is very weak, and the majority of epidemiological studies have found a null relationship between cholesterol in foods and CVD incidence.

However, it should also be remembered that intake of foods high in dietary cholesterol are often associated with intake of foods high in saturated fat, so reducing saturated fat intake will in turn reduce the intake of dietary cholesterol.

Table 7.5 Cholesterol content of foods

Content	Foods	Estimated cholesterol/100 g
High	Liver, offal and products with these	230–690
	Egg yolk, mayonnaise	1120
	Fish roes	500–700
	Shellfish	20–200
Moderate	Fat on meat, duck, goose, and cold cuts	100
	Full-fat milk, cheese, butter, cream	14–100
	Pies, cakes, biscuits, and pastries	40–100
Low	Fish	40–50
	Very lean meats, poultry no skin	50–60
	Skimmed milk, low-fat yoghurt	2–5
	Bread	0–20
Cholesterol-free	All vegetables and vegetable oils, nuts	0
	Fruit including avocado and olives	0
	Egg white, meringue, sugar	0

Dietary interventions to improve risk factors

Disease/ condition	Special considerations

Dyslipidaemia	• Reduction of LDL
	  • Decrease saturated fatty acids and *trans* fatty acids
	  • Choose PUFA, MUFA, and soluble fibre
	  • Consider the use of stanol/sterol esters
	  • Weight loss in the overweight and the obese
	• Increasing HDL
	  • Increase physical activity
	  • Weight loss in the overweight and the obese
	  • Improve glycaemic control in diabetics
	  • Moderate alcohol consumption
	  • Smoking cessation
	• Reduction of triglycerides
	  • Increase physical activity
	  • Weight loss in the overweight and obese
	  • Improved glycaemic control
	  • Reduced alcohol consumption
	  • Reduced sugar consumption; replace with soluble fibre
	  • Increase oily fish consumption/supplementation

Blood pressure	• Reduction of salt intake • Reduction of alcohol intake • Increase potassium and calcium intake from fruit and vegetable intake • Weight loss in the overweight and obese • Increase physical activity
Obesity	• Reduce total calorie intake • Increase physical activity • Set realistic weight loss target (10% in 6 months)
Diabetes and impaired glucose tolerance	• Glycaemic control • Referral to dietitian if poorly controlled (hyper or hypo) • Ensure regular intake of low glycaemic index foods • Follow same guidelines as for CVD • Weight loss in the overweight and obese

Chapter 8

Physical activity and exercise

Introduction to exercise programming

The burden of physical inactivity is of growing concern. WHO data estimates around 3% of all disease burden in developed countries is caused by physical inactivity, and up to 24% of CHD is due to levels of physical activity below 2.5 hours of moderate intensity activity per week. It is estimated that approximately 36% of deaths from CHD in men and 38% of deaths in women are due to lack of physical activity.[1] Therefore, structured exercise training as a therapeutic intervention is central to an effective preventive cardiology programme. In addition to the promotion of general physical activity to all individuals, the programme should focus on achieving gains in physical fitness, which are associated with increased aerobic capacity, muscle strength, endurance, and flexibility, for example.

Table 8.1 Key goals for aerobic training, resistance training, and flexibility training[2,3]

Component of fitness	Frequency	Intensity	Time	Type
Cardiovascular	At least 3 times per week	60–75% HRmax 40–60% HRR RPE 12–15	20–60 min	Aerobic
Muscular strength	2–3 times per week	To moderate fatigue	1 set of 10–15 repetitions	8–10 exercises involving major muscle groups
Flexibility	Minimal 2–3 days per week	Stretch to tightness at the end of the range of motion but not to pain	Hold for 15–30 seconds for each stretch, 2–4 repetitions	Static stretching

1 WHO (2006). *Cardiovascular disease.* Geneva: WHO. Available from: http://www.who.int/cardiovascular_diseases/resources/atlas/en/

2 American College of Sports Medicine (2006). *Guidelines for exercise testing and prescription,* (7th edn). Baltimore: Lippincott, Williams and Wilkins.

3 British Association for Cardiac Rehabiltation (BACR) (2007). BACR exercise instructors' manual 3rd edn Human Kinetics, Leeds.

Exercise prescription and physical activity advice

The exercise prescription and physical activity advice for the individual patient should be based on a detailed assessment (see Chapter 4).

Key information required for provision of a safe, effective, and individualized physical activity and exercise plan is outlined in Box 8.1.

Box 8.1 Information required for physical activity planning and exercise prescription (reproduced with permission from the Association of Chartered Physiotherapists in Cardiac Rehabilitation (ACPICR), 2006)[4]

- History and clinical presentation
- Risk stratification
- Functional capacity test
- Medical diagnosis
- Investigations (e.g. diagnosis, electrocardiogram (ECG) exercise test, echocardiogram report, angiogram, medication)
- Symptoms (e.g. angina, orthopnoea, shortness of breath, claudication, palpitations, ankle swelling, dizziness)
- Physical measures
  - heart rate/rhythm
  - blood pressure
  - body mass index (BMI)
  - blood glucose as appropriate
  - waist/hip ratio, waist circumference
  - habitual physical activity
  - functional capacity
- Psychosocial
  - emotional status
  - occupation
  - state of behavioural change
  - readiness to participate in both structured exercise and increased activity within daily living
  - health beliefs
  - perceived barriers to exercise participation
- Other
  - neuromuscular skeletal system
  - functional goals and limitations
  - dietary intake/food habits
  - co-morbidity

With this information, an individual exercise prescription with goals can be developed in partnership with the patient.

4 Association of Chartered Physiotherapists in Cardiac Rehabilitation (ACPICR) (2006). *Standards for the exercise component of Phase III cardiac rehabilitation*. Stevenage: Pear Tree Press.

Delivery of a supervised exercise component

In order to achieve gains in aerobic capacity, individuals should perform structured exercise, primarily focused on cardiovascular conditioning, three times a week. This structured programme should follow key principles, which can be achieved in many ways, for example within a structured supervised exercise class, structured one-to-one, or using a structured home programme. Whichever mode, or often combination of modes (e.g. twice-weekly group-based supervised exercise and once-weekly home-based programme), is employed there is a common philosophy to the exercise programme format, as summarized in Box 8.2.

Box 8.2 The typical format of structured exercise to gain aerobic fitness[3]

- ***Prior to exercise:***
  - pre-exercise screening for contraindications to exercise, changes in clinical status, or medications
  - recording of pre-exercise heart rate and blood pressure where appropriate
- ***Warm-up:***
  - 15 min in length
  - graduated increase in exercise intensity
  - inclusion of pulse raising, mobility, and stretching bodily movements
  - light exercise intensity (approx. 50–55% HR max and/or rating of perceived exertion (RPE) 10–11)
- ***Conditioning phase:***
  - 20–30 min in length
  - cardiovascular endurance
  - an interval approach for the deconditioned patient, progressing to continuous cardiovascular exercise as able
  - moderate exercise intensity (60–75% of HR max and/or 12–13 RPE)
- ***Cool-down:***
  - 10 min in length
  - graduated lowering of intensity, returning heart rate to near pre-exercise levels
  - 15 min post-exercise observation

Pre-exercise screening and induction to supervised exercise

Prior to each exercise session, individuals should be screened for the presence of any exercise contraindications (Box 8.3).

Box 8.3 Contraindications to participation in exercise training

- Unstable angina
- Resting tachycardia
- Resting blood pressure >200 mmHg systolic and >110 mmHg diastolic (or in community settings >180 mmHg systolic and >100 mmHg diastolic)
- A systolic blood pressure that fails to rise or drops on exercise
- Unstable diabetes
- Unstable heart failure
- Current pyrexia

In addition, prior to participating in structured exercise all individuals should have a programme induction. This induction should include, for example:

- Recognizing the signs and symptoms of overexertion.
- How to correctly manage chest pain and or angina.
- Attending with the appropriate medication or medical monitoring equipment, e.g. glyceryl trinitrate (GTN) and glucose testing kit.
- Understanding appropriate exercise intensity.
- Importance of warm-up and cool-down.
- Wearing suitable clothing and footwear.
- Pre- and post-exercise eating and drinking.
- Advising staff on any recent or worrying symptoms and changes in treatment or medication prior to each attendance.
- Pulse rate and blood pressure monitoring.
- The exercise circuit and equipment.
- Monitoring during exercise, i.e. the patient must inform staff of any changes in symptoms during the exercise session.
- Use of RPE.
- The benefits of exercise.
- Introducing an individual home exercise programme.
- Using exercise record sheets and a home activity diary.

The warm-up (ACPICR and BACR recommendations)[4,5]

A warm-up period provides the transition from resting state to a level of intensity which represents conditioning, i.e. the intensity required to stimulate beneficial physiological adaptation. An effective warm-up prepares the body and mind for the more strenuous activities to follow.

It prepares the body and mind by:

- Raising the pulse rate in a graduated and safe way, thereby avoiding abrupt increases in myocardial workload.
- Redistributing blood to active tissues.
- Increasing muscle temperature.
- Stimulating the release of synovial fluid which facilitates joint movement.

- Focusing the participants' attention on the activity ahead.
- Practising the exercises that are to be performed, thus activating the relevant 'neuromuscular pathways'.

The warm-up should;
- Practise the exercises that are to be performed.
- Be longer and more gradual than that for the apparently healthy population. The warm-up should be no less than 15 minutes for individuals with established coronary heart disease.

An extended warm-up increases the ischaemic threshold through gradual vasodilation of the coronary arteries. Coronary blood flow is also enhanced as a result of increasing aortic pressure as the intensity of exercise increases.

To be effective, the warm-up should consist of the following components, which should flow and gradually increase in intensity:
- Mobility exercises: a gradual progression of range-of-motion exercises to stimulate the release of synovial fluid. The mobility exercises should be interspersed with gentle pulse-raising movements.
- Pulse-raising exercises: progressive movements, using the large muscle groups, which are designed to gradually raise the intensity of the myocardial workload. These pulse-raising activities should slowly raise the heart rate to 20 bpm below target heart rate, or if the Rating of Perceived Exertion Scale (RPE) is used to measure intensity, no higher than 2 on the 0–10 scale or 11 on the 6–20 scale (Box 8.10).
- Preparation stretches interspersed with pulse-raising activities, to ensure that there is no significant decrease in heart rate.
- Re-warm to appropriately elevate the heart rate before the more vigorous cardiovascular exercises.

When analysing a warm-up, the following areas are worthy of consideration:
- Were all joints mobilized? Can any joint movements not included be justified?
- Were appropriate pulse-raising movements included?
- Was intensity raised gradually? If so how?
- The control of a group, and the safety and effectiveness of how the participants perform the exercises, is very dependent upon the teaching techniques that the instructor uses. Were teaching points given?
- Were those teaching points relevant and well communicated?
- Was exercise technique reinforced?
- Were alternatives offered to accommodate individual ability?
- Where stretches were included, were they short and preparatory in nature and did they include interspersed pulse-raising moves?
- Are patients encouraged to self-regulate intensity and not paced by external stimuli?

5 British Association for Cardiac Rehabilitation (2008). *A practical approach to physical activity and exercise in the management of cardiovascular disease.* Human Kinetics, Leeds.

Conditioning phase (ACPICR recommendations)[5]

All patients should participate in an individualized, progressive exercise training programme. The exercise programme, which is considered in addition to physical activity recommendations, should be designed to produce a training effect through varying the frequency, duration, intensity, and mode of exercise. The primary aim is to improve the duration and efficiency of exercise and then increase the intensity.

Frequency

In order to improve functional capacity, exercising at least 3 times a week is recommended. The frequency of structured exercise should be at least twice a week for 6–12 weeks.[2,6]

Intensity

- Aerobic, low- to moderate-intensity exercise, designed to match the range of fitness levels, and which can be undertaken safely and effectively in the home or community, is recommended for most patients undergoing exercise training.[2]
- Target heart rate ranges (see Monitoring exercise intensity, below) and/or RPE (see Monitoring exercise intensity, below) should be prescribed for each individual, based on thorough assessment and risk stratification (Table 4.10).
- Exercise effort should be adjusted to ensure that the workload prescribed is achieving the appropriate target heart rating and perceived exertion that has been calculated for each individual.

Type of exercise

- An interval training approach is recommended which aims to gradually progress the duration of aerobic activities.
- Resistance training, particularly with a muscular endurance focus, is associated with maintenance of strength and can be performed safely by most patients.[2]

Duration of exercise

- A duration of 20–30 minutes is recommended for the conditioning period.[2]

Other exercise considerations

- For muscle strength and endurance exercises, the feet should be kept moving, maintaining venous return.
- Sustained isometric exercises that involve breath holding should be avoided due to the risk of rapid increases in blood pressure and rate pressure product.
- Exercises performed lying down should be avoided during the main conditioning phase. When indicated, floor work (e.g. relaxation exercise and stretching) should be carried out after a cool-down period, when the cardiovascular system has recovered.
- Although seated arm exercise above chest height is acceptable, it requires specific adaptation, i.e. accompanied by mild-intensity associated leg work, to ensure that cardiac output is not compromised.

- The exercise prescription should consider muscle balance and posture, ensuring that opposing muscles are targeted and that 'overuse' and 'overload' of any one muscle group is avoided.
- Correct exercise technique and adaptation of exercise for co-morbidities are important.

6 Scottish Intercollegiate Guidelines Network (SIGN) (2002). *Cardiac rehabilitation: a national clinical guideline*. Edinburgh: SIGN. Available at http://www.sign.ac.uk/guidelines/index.html.

The Cool-down (ACPICR recommendations)[4]

The risk of cardiac complications shortly after stopping an exercise session is well documented and a graded cool-down has been found to reduce the incidence of these complications. A graduated cool-down reduces the levels of circulating catecholamines and maintains venous return, thereby reducing the risk of arrhythmias, a hypotensive episode, or ischaemia through underperfusion of the coronary arteries. Cool-down exercise should be the reverse of the warm-up exercises in most respects, and aims to return the cardiorespiratory system gradually to near pre-exercise levels within 10–15 minutes.[2]

All patients should participate in a cool-down period that includes low-intensity activities and muscle stretching to prevent blood pooling in the lower limbs and to enhance venous return (Box 8.4).

Box 8.4 The cool-down

- The duration should be a minimum of 10 minutes.
- Exercise effort should be decreased gradually from the individual's exercise prescription.
- By the end of the cool-down period the heart rate should have returned to near pre-exercise level.
- A heart rate should be recorded after cool-down.
- Patients should be supervised for a minimum of 15 minutes from the end of the cool–down period. This post-exercise supervision time is often combined with group-based heath-promotion workshops, discussions, or stress management and relaxation techniques.

Monitoring exercise intensity

A training effect is usually associated with exercise intensities greater than 60% of heart rate maximum. Exercise intensity therefore needs to be sufficiently high in order to provoke physiological adaptations through an overload principle. However, in this population group safety is paramount and is the primary consideration. Therefore, in some cases, exercise will need to be prescribed at lower intensities; for example, when an exercise tolerance test identifies ischaemia or the patient becomes symptomatic at lower exercise intensities.

Exercise intensity can be monitored using several methods. In clinical practice a combination of methods is usually used, as each method in isolation has limitations. The methods used to monitor exercise intensity in a cardiovascular disease prevention and rehabilitation programme are summarized in Box 8.5.

Box 8.5 Possible methods for monitoring exercise intensity

- Observation for signs of exertion, e.g. pallor, sweatiness, exercise technique, and co-ordination.
- Heart rate during exercise, e.g. via manual palpation or simple hand-held devices or chest straps.
- Rating of perceived exertion using either the Borg 6–20 scale or category ratio (CR) 0–10 scale (see Boxes 8.10 and 8.11).
- Metabolic equivalents (METS).
- Blood lactate concentrations.

Methods for calculating training heart rate[5]

Several methods can be used to estimate training heart rate ranges (THRR). Where a true maximum heart rate is available, usually ascertained from a maximal exercise tolerance test, the most common methods for calculating training heart rate in a cardiovascular disease prevention and rehabilitation programme include the percentage of true maximum and the Karvonen formula.

Percentage of true maximum

This formula assumes access to true observed maximum heart rate. This may be gained by a maximal ECG tolerance test. Exercise intensity is based on assessment findings and risk stratification. Typically, for initial exercise an intensity of 60–75% of the true heart rate maximum (HRmax) is selected in a cardiovascular disease prevention and rehabilitation programme. Once accustomed, the exercise intensities can increase to 80% HRmax, as long as the patient is asymptomatic at these intensities (Box 8.6).

Box 8.6 Working example of percentage true heart rate maximum formula

Patient X (low risk and uncomplicated) achieves a maximum heart rate of 148 during an ECG exercise tolerance test. The intensity of training following assessment has been set at 60–75% of HR maximum.

$$0.6 \times 148 = 89$$
$$0.75 \times 148 = 111$$

Conclusion: training heart rate = 89–111 beats per minute.

Karvonen formula

This method takes into account resting heart rate. The heart rate reserve (HRR) is calculated by the difference between resting and maximal heart rate (simply the reserve of heart beats required between rest and maximal exertion). This formula again assumes access to a true observed maximum heart rate. This formula is advantageous in that it accounts for the individual's resting heart rate. A percentage of this is selected based on the assessment findings, noting that 40–60% of HRR is equivalent to 60–75% of maximum heart rate (Box 8.7).

Box 8.7 How to calculate training heart rate using the Karvonen formula

STEP1: Heart rate reserve (HRR) is calculated:
HRR = maximum heart rate – resting heart rate
STEP 2: Training intensity is selected and calculated, i.e. 40–60% HRR
STEP 3: Resting heart rate is added back to HRR percentage

For example: patient X (low risk and uncomplicated) has a resting heart rate of 55 and achieves a maximum heart rate of 148 during ECG exercise test. The intensity of training following assessment has been set at 40–60% of HRR.

STEP 1: Calculation of HRR = 148 – 55= 93
STEP 2: Selection of % of HRR

$$40\% \text{ of HRR} = 0.40 \times 93 = 37$$
$$60\% \text{ of HRR} = 0.60 \times 93 = 56$$

STEP 3: Add resting heart rate =

$$37 + 55 = 92$$
$$56 + 55 = 111$$

Conclusion: training heart rate = 92–111 beats per minute.

Where a true maximum heart rate is not available, the most common methods for calculating training heart rate in a cardiovascular disease prevention and rehabilitation programme include the age-adjusted heart rate maximum and age-adjusted Karvonen formula.

For patients taking chronotropic medications (e.g. beta-blockers) this has to be adjusted for in the calculation. Anecdotally, an adjustment of between 20 and 40 beats is typically applied.

Age-adjusted formula

Where an HRmax has not been individually established, it may be estimated using the formula 220 bpm – age (years). This estimation relies on the principle that maximum heart rate declines by approximately 10 beats per decade. This formula uses a predicted maximum heart rate based on age (220 – age). However, there is a standard deviation of ±10 bpm and therefore this is a useful estimate (Box 8.8).

Box 8.8 Working example of age-adjusted heart rate maximum formula

Patient X (low risk and uncomplicated) is 65 years old, not beta-blocked, and has no available exercise tolerance test (ETT) data. The intensity of training following assessment has been set at 60–75% of HRmax.

Age-adjusted HRmax = 220 – age (220 – 65 = 155)

$$0.6 \times 155 = 93$$
$$0.75 \times 155 = 116$$

Conclusion: training heart rate = 93–116 beats

Patient X (low risk and uncomplicated) is 65 years old, taking beta-blockade therapy, and has no available ETT data. The intensity of training following assessment has been set at 60–75% of HR maximum.

Age-adjusted HRmax = 220 – age-adjustment for beta-blockade therapy

$$220 - 65 - 30 = 125$$
$$0.6 \times 125 = 75$$
$$0.75 \times 125 = 94$$

Conclusion: training heart rate = 75–94 beats per minute.

Age-adjusted Karvonen formula

Where HRmax has not been individually established, it may be estimated using the formula 220 bpm – age (years). With the addition of this step, the HRR can then be applied as above, where the difference between the age-predicted maximum and resting heart rate is calculated (Box 8.9).

Box 8.9 How to calculate training heart rate using the age-adjusted Karvonen formula

STEP1: Age-adjusted maximum predicted heart rate is calculated
STEP 2: Heart rate reserve (HRR) is calculated:
HRR = predicted maximum heart rate – resting heart rate
STEP 3: Training intensity is selected and calculated, i.e. 40–60% HRR
STEP 4: Resting heart rate is added back to HRR percentage

For example: patient X, a 50-year-old male (low risk and uncomplicated) has a resting heart rate of 55 and has not undergone a maximal ECG exercise test. The intensity of training following assessment has been set at 40–60% of HRR. He is on beta-blockade therapy.

STEP 1: Calculation predicted age-adjusted heart rate maximum = 220 – age adjustment for beta-blockade therapy

$$220 - 50 - 30 = 140$$

STEP 2: Calculation of HRR = (HRmax – HRrest) = 140 – 55= 85
STEP 3: Selection of % of HRR

$$40\% \text{ of HRR} = 0.40 \times 85 = 34$$
$$60\% \text{ of HRR} = 0.60 \times 85 = 50$$

STEP 4: Add resting heart rate =

$$34 + 55 = 89$$
$$50 + 55 = 105$$

Conclusion: training heart rate = 89–105 beats per minute.

Rating of perceived exertion

In a preventive cardiology programme, intensity of exercise is commonly assessed using either the 6–20 Borg Scale or 0–10 category ratio (CR) scale; 12–14 or 3–4 on Borg's RPE and CR-10 scales, respectively, concur with 60–75% of maximal target heart rate ranges.[7]

7 Borg, G. (1998). *Borg's perceived exertion and pain scales*. Human Kinetics, Champaign, Illinois.

Box 8.10 Borg Rating of perceived exertion (RPE) scale®

6	No exertion at all
7	Extremely light
8	
9	Very light
10	
11	Light
12	
13	Somewhat hard
14	
15	Hard (heavy)
16	
17	Very hard
18	
19	Extremely hard
20	Maximal exertion

In order to ensure that the Borg RPE Scale® is used correctly, the following principles should be followed:

- The scale should be correctly administered (Borg, G. 1998, Borg's Perceived Exertion and Pain Scales, Human Kinetics).
- The patient should be familiarized with using the scale.
- Standardised instructions should be used (Box 8.11)
- The patient should demonstrate a clear understanding of the instructions.
- The scale should be in view at all times.
- Rating of exertion should be asked at the time of exercise and not on reflection.
- The focus should be on the descriptors and not the numbers.
- The patient should not be instructed where on the scale to work initially, as this sets preconceived expectations.
- The patient should experience several anchor points in order to understand the perception of 'somewhat hard' compared to 'light'.
- Once the patient demonstrates consistently that he or she can reliably match their perceived exertion to other objective measures, such as heart rate or METs, then there is less need to monitor heart rate and RPE can be the primary focus.

Box 8.11 Instructions to the Borg RPE Scale®

During the work we want you to rate your perception of exertion i.e. how heavy and strenuous the exercise feels to you and how tired you are. The perception of exertion is mainly felt as strain and fatigue in your muscles and as breathlessness, or aches in the chest. All work requires some effort, even if this is only minimal. This is true also if you only move a little e.g. walking slowly.

Use this scale from 6 to 20, with 6 meaning 'No exertion at all' and 20 meaning 'maximal exertion'.

6 'No exertion at all', means that you don't feel any exertion whatsoever e.g. no muscle fatigue, no breathlessness or difficulties breathing.

9 'Very light' exertion, as taking a shorter walk at your own pace.

13 'A 'Somewhat hard' work, but it still feels OK to continue.

15 'It is 'hard' and tiring, but continuing isn't terribly difficult.

17 'Very hard'. This is very strenuous work. You can still go on, but you really have to push yourself and you are very tired.

19 'An 'extremely' strenuous level. For most people this is the most strenuous work they have ever experienced.

Try to appraise your feeling of exertion and fatigue as spontaneously and as honestly as possible, without thinking about what the actual physical load is. Try not to underestimate and not to overestimate your exertion. It's your own feeling of effort and exertion that is important, not how this compares with other people's. Look at the scale and the expressions and then give a number. Use any number you like on the scale, not just one of those with an explanation behind it.

Any questions?

Box 8.12 Borg CR10 Scale®

0	Nothing at all	
0.3		
0.5	Extremely weak	Just noticeable
0.7		
1	Very weak	
1.5		
2	Weak	Light
2.5		
3	Moderate	
4		
5	Strong	Heavy
6		
7	Very strong	
8		
9		
10	Extremely strong	"Maximal"
11		
●	Absolute maximum	Highest possible

Note that a license is required to use Borg CR10 scale®

Metabolic equivalents (METs)

The metabolic equivalent (MET) is a means of expressing energy usage/expenditure. One metabolic equivalent (1 MET) is defined as the amount of energy required to serve the body's energy needs at rest. In absolute terms this equals an oxygen uptake (VO_2) of 3.5 ml/kg of body mass/minute (3.5 ml kg^{-1} min^{-1}). Hence, in relative terms, energy expenditure can be described in multiples of resting energy requirements. For example, if a person is walking and has a $V\dot{O}_2$ of 7 ml/kg of body mass/ minute this would equate to 2 METs, as twice the energy requirement of rest is being utilized.[5]

This oxygen consumption expressed as a multiple of resting rate (METs) has been established for many activities[13] and is a useful way to compare relative energy requirements of activities irrespective of the weight of an individual. The MET values for some activities of daily living and for some popular leisure-time activities are summarized in Table 8.2.

Exercise intensity may also be regulated by prescribing activities on the basis of their known MET values. As an example, if an individual can walk for 20 minutes at 3 mph at 70% of his/her THRR and perceives the level of exertion required as 13 on the Borg 6–20 scale, one can safely assume that other activities of comparable MET values will also be well tolerated and represent a cardiovascular training stimulus.[14] So if this individual can comfortably achieve 3–3.5 METs, the energy cost for walking at 3 mph (Table 8.2), all activities of 3.5 METs or less should theoretically also be achievable.

METs are very useful when advising on activities. Many patients ask questions such as 'Can I play golf?' and in these circumstances METs prove to be a useful tool. Advice can be based on ascertaining activities that are currently achievable; for example, can you climb the stairs? If the patient says that he/she climbs the stairs and rates this as light, then theoretically golf (which equates to between 4 and 7 METs) is also achievable, as it is associated with similar energy requirements.

METs can be used in prescribing exercise. By ascertaining an individual's current MET value that is associated with evoking training, i.e. usually exercise intensities greater than 60% HRmax or 13 on the 6–20 RPE scale (see Box 8.10), the same intensity can be prescribed using equipment; for example, by setting a treadmill to a particular speed, a cycle ergometer to selected watts, or a metronome stepping rate on a step block of a known height. All these exercises can be manipulated to produce similar workloads.

Table 8.2 Approximate energy requirements in METs for tasks of daily living/hobbies/sports[2,5,8]

Task	METS (minimum)	METS (maximum)
Walking 2 mph	2	3
Dressing	2	3
Bathing	2	3
Washing dishes	2	3
Ironing	2	4
Dusting	2	4
Bed making	2	6
Walking 3 mph	3	3.5
Shower	3	4
Sexual intercourse	3	5
Raking leaves	3	5
Housework general	3	4
Cleaning windows	3	4
Walking upstairs	4	7
Washing car	6	7
Sailing (small)	2	5
Cycling 5 mph	2	3
Croquet	2	3.5
Fishing (boat)	2	4
Billiards	2	3
Hand drilling	2.7	4.6
Ballroom dancing	4	5
Golf (carrying clubs)	4	5
Swimming (slow)	4	5
Swimming (crawl)	9	10

8 Ainsworth, B. E. (2002). *The compendium of physical activities tracking guide*. Prevention Research Center, Norman J. Arnold School of Public Health, University of South Carolina.

Health and safety[4]

There should be a local protocol to ensure the health and safety[16] of all patients and staff when delivering a supervised exercise component as part of a cardiovascular disease prevention and rehabilitation programme. The safety of patients during a supervised exercise component will be optimized with accurate risk stratification assessment (Table 4.10), appropriate exercise prescription, and effective induction (see Pre-exercise screening and an induction to supervised exercise, above). These should be performed by appropriately trained members of staff and a safe exercise environment should be maintained.

Staffing

Each exercise session should be appropriately staffed:

- There should be a minimum of two appropriately trained health professionals present at all supervised exercise sessions.
- The ratio of staff to patients should depend on the risk stratification of the patients and level of supervision required by the individuals within the group.
- The ACPICR current recommended ratio is 1:5.
- The number of staff should be increased for more complex patient presentation.
- Staff supervising exercise testing and training sessions should have had immediate life support (ILS) training.

Screening and management

- All patients should be screened prior to each exercise session to ensure that they do not have contraindications to exercise.
- All patients should have an exercise induction, be observed during the exercise session and for 15 minutes after cessation of the cool-down component.

Venue and environment

- Appropriate resuscitation equipment, including a defibrillator, with at least one member of staff trained to use it, and access to advanced life support services should be readily available at every supervised exercise session.
- There should be evidence of a locally agreed protocol for medical emergencies during an exercise session.
- There should be a written emergency procedure clearly displayed in the exercise area.
- Resuscitation equipment must be maintained in accordance with local protocols.
- The temperature should be maintained between 65 and 72°F (18–23°C) and humidity at 65%.[2,5,4]
- Drinking water and glucose supplements should be available at all times.
- The size of the exercise area should allow for safe placement and appropriate space around equipment and safe patient movement around the exercise room.

Home exercise programming

- Often formal exercise classes are not frequent enough (i.e. three times per week) to provoke a training effect, and therefore should be supplemented with a structured home-based exercise programme.
- A home programme needs to be designed on an individual basis. It must be realistic and achievable.
- It should follow the FITT (frequency, intensity, time, type) principle, aiming for three times per week of moderate-intensity sustained aerobic activity.
- The home programme should be sensitive to each individual's values and beliefs. Concerns and barriers should be explored.
- Information about the benefits of physical activity, RPE, and monitoring intensity should be provided.
- Goals should be set appropriately, taking into account habitual, past, and present activity levels. Goals should be reviewed on a regular basis.
- Activity diaries, regular reviews, and record keeping are a useful adjunct.

Key principles

The activity or exercise should be of moderate intensity. For example:
- Sustained, rhythmic movements such as brisk walking.
- Feeling warm and slightly out of breath.
- A perceived exertion of 11–14 on the Borg scale.
- 'The talk test'—able to sustain a conversation.

People should be physically active at least 30 minutes a day, five times a week. This can be accumulated in bouts of 10–15 minutes for the low-capacity or sedentary individual.

Endurance training should be performed three times a week. This activity should aim to improve cardiorespiratory fitness and:
- Be aerobic in nature.
- Include activities of daily living for the low-capacity or sedentary patient.
- Include structured exercise sessions where appropriate.

Local facilities, specialist schemes, experts, activities, and facilities available in the local community should be available to individuals to assist them in sustaining activity in the longer term.

Home walking programme designed to gain cardiorespiratory fitness[5]

Warm-up:	A slow walk of 15 minutes
Main component:	Brisk walking for as long as 20–30 minutes, using an interval approach where appropriate. In an interval approach the patient is encouraged to slow down on achievement of a 'somewhat hard' RPE (13 on the 6–20 RPE scale or 4 on the 0–10 CR scale) and then speed up again on achievement of 'light' RPE (11 on the 6–20 scale or 2 on the 0–10 CR scale) (see Boxes 8. 10 and 8.11).

Cool-down: A slow walk of 10 minutes, where the patient feels that by the end he/she has returned to near pre-exercise state before stopping.

Home structured circuit programme designed to gain cardiorespiratory fitness[5]

Warm-up

A minimum of 15 minutes, gradually increasing range of motion at all major joints and slowly increasing the intensity of pulse-raising moves. This allows the body to prepare for activity but, most importantly, it gives the heart muscle time to increase its blood supply so it can respond safely to the extra physical demands. Short stretches for muscles that are to be challenged can be included between pulse-raising movements towards the end.

Circuit

The circuit consists of cardiovascular (CV) exercises and active recovery (AR) exercises. AR exercises are designed to provide rest intervals between cardiorespiratory work stations.

Level 1 starts with alternating minute of CV exercise followed by 12–15 repetitions on an AR exercise. Duration of cardiorespiratory work is increased over the weeks.

Level 1: 5 CV and 5 AR alternating stations (10 minutes CV)
Level 2: 6 CV and 4 AR (12 minutes CV)
Level 3: 7 CV and 3 AR (14 minutes CV)
Level 4: 8 CV and 2 AR (16 minutes CV)
Level 5: 10 CV (20 minutes CV)

The participant chooses the position of the AR station in the circuit from Level 2 onwards, dependent on fatigue levels and personal functional needs.

Exercise 1 (CV)

Walk up and down the hallway for 2 minutes. Progress to walking faster, then alternate walking with jogging.

Exercise 2 (AR)

Bicep curls with empty water bottles. Fill the bottles with water or sand to increase resistance; 12–15 repetitions—keep the feet moving.

Exercise 3 (CV)

Forward or backward lunges for 2 min. Progress by increasing range of movement and/or adding bigger arm movements.

Exercise 4 (AR)

Wall press-ups, 12–15 repetitions. Progress by taking the body further away from the wall and/or doing the exercise more slowly. Alternative: use a resistance band for chest press.

Exercise 5 (CV)

Side taps/alternate side taps for 2 minutes. Progress by increasing range of movement and/or adding graduated arm movements.

Exercise 6 (AR)

Upright row, with empty water bottles/light weights or a resistance band. Fill the bottles with water or sand to increase resistance or use a stronger band; 12–15 repetitions.

Exercise 7 (CV)

Step on and off the bottom step of the stairs for 2 mins. Progress by climbing/descending the stairs.

Exercise 8 (AR)

Seated-low row with resistance band firmly anchored around the feet, or use bottles with water or sand to increase resistance; 12–15 repetitions.

Exercise 9 (CV)

Hamstring curls for 2 minutes. Progress by increasing range of movement and/or adding graduated arm movements.

Exercise 10 (AR)

Lateral (or front) arm raising. Fill bottles with water or sand to increase resistance; 12–15 repetitions.

Cool-down

Gradually lower the intensity of the CV movements and/or walk around the house or garden at a low intensity (10 minutes).

With thanks for the contributions of the British Association for Cardiac Rehabilitation and the Association of Chartered Physiotherapists in Cardiac Rehabilitation to this chapter.

Chapter 9

Principles of managing weight loss

The causes of obesity

Prevalence of obesity

Obesity is a growing problem throughout the world. In the UK the prevalence of obesity has trebled in 20 years. It is associated with increased mortality and morbidity. It is caused by a combination of poor, high-calorie diets and a sedentary lifestyle, on top of a possible genetic disposition of some individuals to be more susceptible to weight gain.

Prevention of obesity

Prevention of obesity is a key, long-term public health goal. This includes all stages of prevention:

- Prevention of weight gain in subjects of healthy weight.
- Prevention of further weight gain in overweight and obese subjects.
- Prevention of weight regain following successful weight loss.

Diet and physical activity are no doubt the main key components in the prevention of weight gain.

Causes of obesity

Environmental

- Global increases in obesity are related to urban and economic development, through increased availability of food and energy-saving developments such as cars and machinery, and a reduction in manual occupations.
- Increase in portion sizes supplied by manufacturers.
- Advertising.

Behavioural (common)

- High-fat, energy-dense diet with a sedentary lifestyle are critical behaviours associated with obesity.
- High-fat diets are more energy dense, therefore for the same volume of food more energy is consumed when compared to carbohydrate.
- Physical activity helps to attenuate the rate of weight gain rather than accelerate weight loss.

Metabolic

- Defect in the metabolic control of appetite.
- Lower metabolic rate unlikely to be a cause (weight gain increases energy requirements).
- This is an area of much research.

Genetic (rare)

- Differences in leptin production or regulation.
- Monogenic disorders in the *ob* gene, pro-opiomelaninocortin processing, or mutations in the MC4 receptor gene, which cause severe obesity.
- Polymorphisms in other genes have less dramatic effects.

Central obesity

Central obesity is an important predictor of CVD and diabetes. It is directly related to the amount of visceral fat. The distribution of excess fat around the middle is thought to be more important than total fat. The waist to hip measure is the best predictor of CVD risk, but waist circumference is a convenient measure of abdominal adipose tissue and correlates almost as well with CVD risk factors. Ideal levels are shown in Boxes 4.4 and 4.5.

Table 9.1 Factors that may protect or cause overweight and obesity (source: WHO/FAO, 2003)[1]

Evidence	Decreases risk	Increases risk
Good	Regular PA High-fibre diet	Sedentary High-fat energy-dense diet
Probable	Environments promoting healthy choices for children Breastfeeding	++ marketing of energy-dense and fast food Adverse social and economic conditions High-sugar drinks
Possible	Low glycaemic index diets	Large portions + Eating out of home Rigid eating patterns
Insufficient	Increased frequency of eating	Alcohol

Box 9.1 Abnormalities associated with obesity and central obesity

A cluster of the following substantially increases the risk of CVD
- Insulin resistance
- Hyperinsulinaemia
- Glucose intolerance
- Type 2 diabetes
- Poor lipid profile (raised TAG; raised, small, dense LDL and HDL)
- Hypertension
- Endothelial dysfunction
- Impaired fibrinolysis and increased susceptibility to thrombosis
- Low chronic inflammation state
- Osteoarthritis
- Gout
- Sleep apnoea
- Breathlessness
- Gall bladder disease
- Cancers (colon, kidney, prostrate, breast, and endometrial)
- Infertility
- Increased anaesthetic risk

1 WHO/FAO (2003). *Diet, nutrition and the prevention of chronic diseases.* WHO Technical report series 916. Geneva: WHO.

The principles of energy balance

The concept of energy balance is the most important concept to understand for long-term weight management. If the energy you take in from your food and drink equals the energy you use up each day (metabolic rate and physical activity), your weight will remain stable. Altering this balance will lead to either weight gain or weight loss.

KEY MESSAGE FOR MAINTENANCE OR WEIGHT CHANGES

ENERGY IN = ENERGY OUT: WEIGHT STABLE

ENERGY IN GREATER THAN ENERGY OUT: WEIGHT GAIN

ENERGY IN LESS THAN ENERGY OUT: WEIGHT LOSS

It does not take very much to gain or lose weight. Having only 100 extra calories each day can add up to 10 pounds (4.5 kg) of weight gain in one year.

Having an energy deficit of 500 calories/day will usually result in about 1 pound (0.5 kg) weight loss each week. A deficit of 1000 calories/day will result in a 2 pound (1 kg) weight loss each week.

This deficit in energy balance will result in weight loss no matter what the weight of the individual was at the start, or the type of diet consumed.

Research has shown that long-term success has much less to do with the type of diet than the perseverance of the participants.

Characteristics of those who are able to maintain weight loss

- Make long-term changes to their lifestyle, not just their diet.
- Monitor their progress (weight, waist, check food records, and physical activity levels).
- Set realistic goals.
- Become used to eating less.
- Healthy eating habits.
- Physically active.
- Focus on long-term goal.

Obtaining information on energy intake and dietary habits

It is well known that obese people tend to underestimate their dietary intake. This obviously confounds analysis of dietary intake, but it does not invalidate invaluable information on dietary habits (qualitative rather than quantitative). Particular areas of discussion with patients should cover the following:

- Meal patterns (regular meals and/or snacks).
- Food and drink preferences.
- Food preparation—who is responsible for shopping and cooking?
- Work facilities—canteen, kitchen, need to eat out.
- Facilities at home.
- Interest in food and drink.
- Weekend/days off—how do these differ?
- Explore possibilities of binge, night, or emotional eating.
- Portion sizes—using photographs or models can be helpful.
- Alcohol intake.
- Reasons for eating (hunger, boredom, comfort, stress, tiredness, social).
- Eating out or takeaways.

Setting targets for losing weight

Rationale for weight loss

It is essential to try to establish why people want to lose weight. The level of motivation a person has often collates with their level of success. The following questions may help identify how motivated a person is:

- Why do you want to lose weight?
  - For health/appearance/emotional reasons?
- Have you tried to lose weight before?
  - What was successful or unsuccessful?
- What support networks do you have in place?
  - Who can support you or who will not be supportive?
- How willing are you to address your physical activity levels?
  - Refer to physical activity section.
- What are the costs and benefits of weight loss?
  - What you have to give up or do to achieve the weight loss goal; does this outweigh the benefits of weight loss?
- What are the potential barriers to implementing the necessary changes?
  - Work patterns/time/family pressures.
- Are you ready and willing to make the necessary changes?
  - Have the barriers and relapse strategies been identified and solutions thought about?
  - What is the patient's stage of change? (See Chapter 5.)

Stage of change and motivation

These questions not only help to identify the level of someone's motivation but may also help to identify their stage of change. Changing behaviours and maintaining them is the key to successful treatment of obesity. Further information on behaviour change can be found in Chapter 5.

Target weights

Many people have an 'ideal weight' in their mind when they set out to lose weight. There are also guidelines set out by the WHO using BMI. It is important to set realistic targets.

Research has shown that individuals who are overweight or obese can vastly improve their health by losing as little as 10% of their present body weight.[2]

Box 9.2 Benefits of a 10 kg weight loss in a 100 kg subject

Mortality	20–25% decrease in premature mortality
Blood pressure	10 mmHg decrease in systolic pressure 20 mmHg decrease in diastolic pressure
Lipids	10% decrease in total cholesterol 15% decrease in LDL cholesterol 8% increase in HDL cholesterol 30% decrease in triglycerides
Diabetes	Reduces risk of developing type 2 diabetes by 50% 30–50% decrease in elevated blood glucose 15% decrease in HbA1c

Dietary and physical activity targets

When setting dietary targets, try to ensure they are measurable and realistic. Make sure the goals are clearly defined in terms of what, when, and how.

For example

- I will skip desert every day, I will choose a low-calorie sandwich 3 days a week, I will walk the dog for 1 hour 3 days a week.

Setting these short-term, measurable goals, enables people to feel successful easily and quickly. These short-term goals are the small steps that are required to meet the longer-term goals.

It is important that people who are trying to lose weight recognize and reward themselves on achieving these goals, but at the same time plan the next goals to be achieved.

2 SIGN. Obesity in Scotland. Integrating Prevention with weight management. A National Clinical Guideline recommended for use in Scotland. 1996.

How to reduce calorie intake

For weight loss to occur there needs to be an energy deficit. A deficit of 500 kcal/day can result in approximately 1 pound (0.5 kg) weight loss each week.

The most important thing to work out with the patient is what dietary method is most likely to have a positive outcome. Everyone is an individual, so different dietary plans work for different people. There are many diets on the market, but they all have the same overall aim: to create an energy deficit through calorie counting, portion control, meal replacements, nutrient combining, or set meal plans.

The most difficult part of losing weight is actually maintaining that loss. Poor eating habits and portion sizes are learned habits, we can re-learn these. It is essential that the patient implements a healthy lifestyle to enable maintenance of the weight loss achieved.

Different calorie reduction strategies

Swapping of food

By replacing high-calorie foods with lower-calorie foods.

For example

- Vanilla ice-cream for a fruit sorbet — 139 kcal saved
- Caesar salad or salad with light dressing — 140 kcal saved
- ½ cup fried rice to ½ cup steamed rice — 53 kcal saved
- Café latte to cappuccino — 80 kcal saved
- 100 g full-fat cream cheese to low-fat cream cheese — 144 kcal saved

This method is often effective for those people who have a routine. This means it is relatively easy to identify the foods or drinks that can be swapped to reduce their calorie intake enough to promote weight loss.

Reduction of total intake

This is by simply reducing the overall intake of the food normally eaten. Care needs to be taken with this method, particularly if the overall dietary pattern is not healthy. Although reducing the intake will aid weight loss, the maintenance of this may be more difficult if the overall pattern is not healthy.

For example

- 2 slices of toast rather than 3
- 3 tablespoons of rice rather than 4
- 3 oz of meat (deck of playing cards) rather than 6 oz (2 decks)
- 1 teaspoon of mayonnaise rather than 1 dessertspoon

This approach often works well for people who have no routine and are on the go a lot. But focus must also be placed on ways of improving the diet to bring it in line with the cardioprotective recommendations (see Chapter 7, What is a cardioprotective diet?).

Changing the proportion of food groups in the diet

This method may help patients to reduce their calorie intake by changing the proportion of food groups within the diet. As shown in Fig. 9.1, it encourages the reduction of protein and carbohydrate foods and replaces them with fruit and vegetables, so the total volume remains the same. This will also help to encourage a healthy balance.

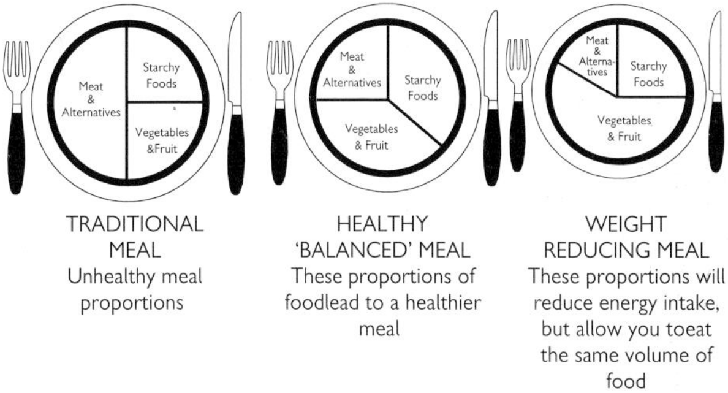

Fig. 9.1 Proportion of food groups in the diet. Reproduced with permission from the Dietetic Department, Imperial College Healthcare NHS Trust.

With this method the tip is to put the vegetables on the plate first, followed by starchy food and then the protein food. This idea needs to be applied to all meals. The patient should draw their plate next to the meal described in the diary.

Low glycaemic diet

Weight loss or satiety have been shown to be no different between low and high glycaemic diets (see Chapter 7, Glycaemic index).

High protein/low carbohydrate diets

These are the diets described by the Dr Atkin's 'diet revolution'. Initial weight loss is due to glycogen and water losses. Protein induces high satiety and therefore causes reduced intake. A systematic review concluded that there was insufficient evidence for or against this approach. There are no long-term data on CVD risk factors.

Hidden calories

Awareness of hidden calories in food and drinks is essential. Foods may look or sound healthy, but when looking at the contents there are often high levels of fat or sugar. For example, muesli bars with yoghurt, 98% fat-free biscuits/cakes, light butter. Therefore it is essential to read the nutritional information on the product. Using the per 100 g/100 ml column enables comparison of products.

	per 100g		
	Low	**Moderate**	**High**
Total fat/ sugar	<3 g	2–20 g	>20 g
Saturated fat	<1.5 g	1.5–5 g	>5 g

Other interventions for obesity

Pharmaceutical support for obesity

Diet, physical activity and exercise play a central role in preventing obesity and are the first-line treatment for the condition. But many patients may benefit from drugs to help them lose weight.

What obesity drugs can do

- Improve weight loss over and above that achieved by lifestyle changes alone.
- Help with maintaining weight loss.
- Improve risk factor profiles for CVD.
- May help patients to learn which foods are more suitable due to side effects, e.g. orlistat (Xenical®).

How do they work?

They either work through appetite suppression, inducing malabsorption, or by thermogenesis to increase energy expenditure. The best outcome occurs when they are given in conjunction with diet, exercise, and behaviour therapy.

Obesity drugs available

No trials have compared the drugs directly. Initial choice should be based on patient preference, CV risk, and side-effects.

Orlistat

- Lipase inhibitor that generates malabsorption of 30% of dietary fat.
- 20% of patients achieve 5% weight loss.
- Outcome is better when lifestyle support is provided.
- Reduces LDL, blood pressure and diabetes incidence. Therefore it is the first choice for those with CVD, at high risk of developing diabetes, or high LDL.
- Avoid in those with chronic diarrhoea.
- Patients will need to follow a low-fat diet, as high-fat foods may cause diarrhoea.

Sibutramine

- Causes satiety enhancement by inhibiting reuptake of noradrenaline (norepinephrine) and serotonin.
- 34% reached 5% weight loss, but higher with lifestyle support.
- Increases HDL and useful in those who snack.
- Not licensed for use in those with CVD, raised BP, or tachycardia.
- Main side-effects: dry mouth, constipation, headaches, and dizziness.

Surgery for weight loss

The most common stomach surgery is vertical banded gastroplication. The more invasive, gastric bypass is now much less used. Other approaches include liposuction and intragastric balloon treatment, but these are ineffective and rarely used.

A multidisciplinary team is essential for this type of obesity treatment. The team usually includes:

- Physician/surgeon
- Dietitian/nutritionist
- Clinical psychologist
- Nurse

Morbidly obese people have a high anesthetic risk, and respiratory problems can require intensive care (ITU) support. Assessment must ensure that the risk of the surgery does not outweigh the outcome. As well as the normal/common problems associated with surgery, these subjects may also have nutritional, emotional, and psychiatric problems.

Most of the weight loss following surgery occurs during the first 2 years, after which weight regain occurs, although this is still significantly lower than the original weight (40–65% of preoperative weight after 5 years; 16.7% after 10 years).[3–5]

3 National Institute for Health and Clinical Excellence. (2002). *The clinical effectiveness and cost effectiveness of surgery for people with morbid obesity*. Technology Appraisal No. 46. London: NICE.

4 Kral, J.G. (1992). Overview of surgical techniques for treating obesity. *American Journal of Clinical Nutrition*, **55**, 552–5.

5 Sjostrom, L. (2000). Surgical intervention as a strategy for treatment of obesity. *Endocrine*, **13**, 213–30.

Chapter 10

Blood pressure, lipids and glucose

Lifestyle modification and the management of blood pressure

An emphasis on lifestyle modification is important in effective blood pressure management pressure for the following reasons:

- Reduction in the need for pharmacological intervention.
- Reduction in the need for combination therapy.
- Beneficial in terms of reducing overall cardiovascular risk.

Key lifestyle recommendations are outlined in Box 10.1.

Box 10.1 Lifestyle recommendations for reducing blood pressure

- Reduction in salt consumption <6 g/day.
- Reduced total fat and saturated fat intake.
- Consumption of five portions of fruit and vegetables/day.
- Weight reduction.
- Increased physical activity.
- Limitation in alcohol consumption.

Diet

- The DASH study[1] showed that a diet high in fruit and vegetables and low-fat dairy products, and low in saturated fat, total fat, and cholesterol, produced a striking reduction in BP (11.4 and 5.5 mmHg for systolic and diastolic measurements, respectively).
- Reduced salt intake lowers blood pressure in those with both high and normal blood pressure levels (–4.8/–2.5 and –1.9/–1.1 mmHg, respectively).[2] Current guidelines limit salt intake to <6 g/day.
- Increased potassium consumption will also have an antihypertensive effect, with consumption of foods high in potassium preferable to potassium supplementation.[3]
- There is some evidence to suggest that increased monounsaturated fat and protein may have a BP-lowering effect, but further research is warranted and this is not routinely recommended.

Alcohol

Observational studies have confirmed a clear relationship between high alcohol intake and elevated BP. Furthermore, reduction in alcohol consumption can reduce systolic and diastolic BP levels by –3.1 mmHg and –2.04 mmHg, respectively.[4] Alcohol intake should be limited to <21 units per week (men) and <14 units/week (women) (see Table 7.1, p.126).

Weight loss

Studies consistently show that weight loss lowers blood pressure and this effect may occur even before or without achievement of an ideal body weight.[5]

Physical activity

Regular exercise lowers BP and, interestingly, this effect is independent of changes in body weight.[6]

1 Appel, L.J., Moore, T.J., Obarzanek, E., *et al.* (1997). A clinical trial of the effects of dietary patterns on blood pressure. DASH Collaborative Research Group. *New England Journal of Medicine*, **336**(16), 1117–24.

2 Cutler, J.A., Follmann, D., and Allender, P.S. (1997). Randomized trials of sodium reduction: an overview. American Journal of Clinical Nutrition, **65**(2 Suppl), 643S–51S.

3 Whelton, P.K., He, J., Cutler, J.A., *et al.* Effects of oral potassium on blood pressure. Meta-analysis of randomized controlled clinical trials. *Journal of the American Medical Association*, **277**(20), 1624–32.

4 Xin, X., He, J., Frontini, M.G., Ogden, L.G., Motsamai, O.I., and Whelton, P.K. (2001). Effects of alcohol reduction on blood pressure: a meta-analysis of randomized controlled trials. *Hypertension*, **38**(5), 1112–17.

5 Staessen, J., Fagard, R., Lijnen, P., and Amery, A. (1989). Body weight, sodium intake and blood pressure. *Journal of Hypertension Suppl* , **7**(1), S19–S23.

6 Whelton, S.P., Chin, A., Xin, X., and He, J. (2002). Effect of aerobic exercise on blood pressure: a meta-analysis of randomized, controlled trials. *Annals of Internal Medicine,* **136**(7), 493–503.

Treatment protocol for blood pressure

Risk stratification

- The decision to start blood pressure medication depends not only on the blood pressure levels but also on total CVD risk
- The presence of clinically established cardiovascular disease or diabetes markedly increases the risk of cardiovascular events
- People with target organ damage should be managed as 'increased risk'
- People with particularly elevated blood pressure are at sufficiently high CVD risk on the basis of blood pressure levels alone to require blood pressure lowering medication

JES4

Blood pressure targets

- Blood pressure should be reduced to < 140/90 mmHg (and lower if tolerated) in all hypertensive patients who qualify for drug treatment
- In all high risk people, especially those with established CVD and diabetes a blood pressure of 130/80 mmHg is desirable, if feasible

Table 10.1 Management of total CVD risk: blood pressure. In all cases, look for and manage all risk factors. Those with established CVD, diabetes or renal disease are at markedly increased risk and a BP of <130/80 is desirable, if feasible. For all other people, check SCORE risk. Those with target organ damage are managed as 'increased risk' (reproduced from the European Guidelines on CVD Prevention, *European Journal of Cardiovascular Prevention and Rehabilitation* 2007; Vol 14 (suppl 2: S1–S113) ©ESC 2007)

SCORE CVD risk	Normal <130/85	High normal 130–139/85–89	Grade I 140–159/ 90–99	Grade 2 160–179/ 100–109	Grade 3 ≥180/110
Low <1%	Lifestyle advice	Lifestyle advice	Lifestyle advice	Drug therapy if persists	Drug therapy
Mod. 1–4%	Lifestyle advice	Lifestyle advice	+ Consider drug therapy	Drug therapy if persists	Drug therapy
Increased 5-9%	Lifestyle advice	+ Consider drug therapy	Drug therapy	Drug therapy	Drug therapy
Markedly increased ≥10%	Lifestyle advice	+ Consider drug therapy	Drug therapy	Drug therapy	Drug therapy

JBS2

Blood pressure targets

- The optimal blood pressure target in people at high risk of developing CVD is < 140/85 mmHg
- In people with established CVD and diabetes the blood pressure target is < 130/80 mmHg

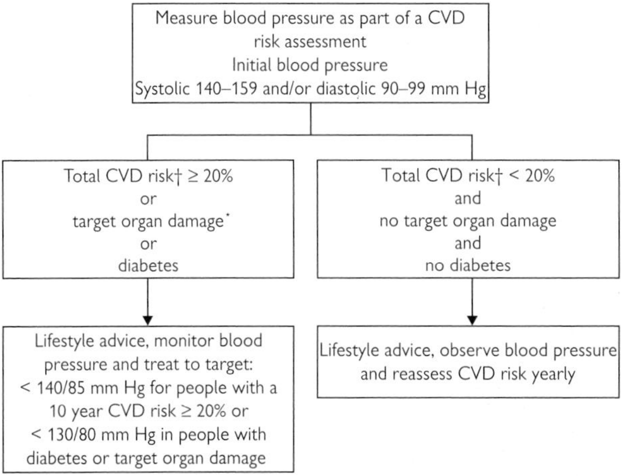

Fig. 10.1 Risk thresholds and targets for blood pressure in adsymptomatic people without CVD. †Assessed with CVD risk chart. Reproduced with permission from British Cardiac Society, British Hypertension Society, Diabetes UK, HEART UK, Primary Care Cardiovascular Society, The Stroke Association. JBS2 (2005) Joint British Societies' guidelines on prevention of cardiovascular disease in clinical practice. *Heart*, 91(Suppl V), V1–V5.

Initiating Drug therapy

The decision with regards to which antihypertensive to be used should be based on several factors including patient characteristics (e.g. ethnicity, age, history of side effects) and medical history and should also try and be in accordance with the national guidelines. (Ref BHS guidelines, ESC guidleines).

Several key facts with regards to antihypertensive therapy should be considered:

1. Lifestyle modification remains very important
2. For the main groups of antihypertensives (e.g. ACE inhibitors, ARBs, diuretics, calcium channel blockers, alpha blockers), each class at its standard dose tends to provide a 9/5 mm Hg blood pressure lowering effect.
3. There is however substantial variation from person to person.

4. Doubling an antihypertensive from half its standard dose to full dose tends to give only a further 20% BP reduction. However, for calcium channel blockers, thiazide diuretics and less so for beta blockers, there is an accompanying rise in the incidence of side effects. This tends not to be the case with ACE inhibitors or ARBs.
5. Monotherapy rarely achieves good blood pressure control. In most patients dual or even triple therapy is required. For each antihypertensive added, one should expect the same BP lowering effect as if that drug was used in isolation.

Which antihypertensive?

Antihypertensive drugs

- ACE inhibitors
- Angiotensin receptor blockers (ARB)
- Diuretics
- β blockers
- Calcium channel blockers
- α blockers

Meta analyses have shown that BP reduction per se, rather than individual classes of drugs is responsible for reduction in cardiovascular risk. Nontheless, in certain individuals one class of antihypertensive may be favoured over another. For more information please read the following references.[1,2] Some key points to remember are:

- Younger patients (<55 years) and Caucasians tend to have higher renin levels relative to older people or those of African descent and so ACE inhibitors/ARBs may be considered first line for the former.
- ACE inhibitors (or ARBs if ACE inhibitor intolerant) should also be used first line in those with established vascular disease.
- Calcium channel blockers and diuretics are better used first line in older patients or those of African descent
- The combination of beta blockers and thiazide diuretics may increase the likelihood of developing diabetes mellitus and should be avoided in those at risk of same (e.g. those with impaired glucose tolerance, obesity, family history etc).

Persistently elevated blood pressure despite treatment

Consider lack of adherence to therapy. It is estimated that up to 50% of patients discontinue taking their antihypertensives at on year. Reasons for this include

- Cost
- Unclear instructions
- Lack of education
- Lack of involvement of patient in planning
- Side effects
- Complexity

1 JBS2 (2005). Joint British Societies' guidelines on prevention of cardiovascular disease in clinical practice. *Heart*, **91**(Suppl 5), v1–v52.

2 Graham, I., Atar, D., Borch-Johnsen, K. *et al.* (2007). European guidelines on cardiovascular disease prevention in clinical practice: full text. Fourth Joint Task Force of the European Society of Cardiology and other Societies on Cardiovascular Disease Prevention in Clinical Practice. *European Journal of Cardiovascular Prevention and Rehabilitation*, **14**(Suppl 2), S1–S113.

Thus, patient education and empowerment is very important in the course of the preventive cardiology programme. The course of the programme also allows sufficient time for drug side effects to emerge and be dealt with either through dose reduction or drug switching.

If a patient is truly adherent to therapy and remains hypertensive on at least three drugs, the white coat effect should be considered. A 24 hour blood pressure monitor showing normal values when the patient is out of the clinical environment will confirm this. If however, blood pressure remains persistently elevated, secondary causes of hypertension should be considered and the patient should be referred for further investigations.

Treatment protocol for lipid management

Risk stratification

- The decision to start lipid lowering medication depends not only on the lipid levels but also on total CVD risk. In all cases, look and manage all risk factors.
- Hyperlipidaemias secondary to other conditions (in particular hypothyroidism, heavy alcohol intake, poorly controlled diabetes) must be excluded before starting treatment, especially with drugs, since often the treatment of secondary hyperlipidaemias can improve blood lipids and no other antilipaemic therapy is necessary.
- Patients with genetic dyslipidaemias such as familial hypercholesterolemia should be referred to specialist evaluation, which might include molecular genetic diagnosis.
- People with particularly elevated total and LDL cholesterol are at sufficiently high CVD risk on the basis of lipid levels alone to require lowering medication.
- The presence of clinically established CVD or diabetes markedly increases the *risk* cardiovascular events.

Table 10.2 Management of total CVD risk–lipids

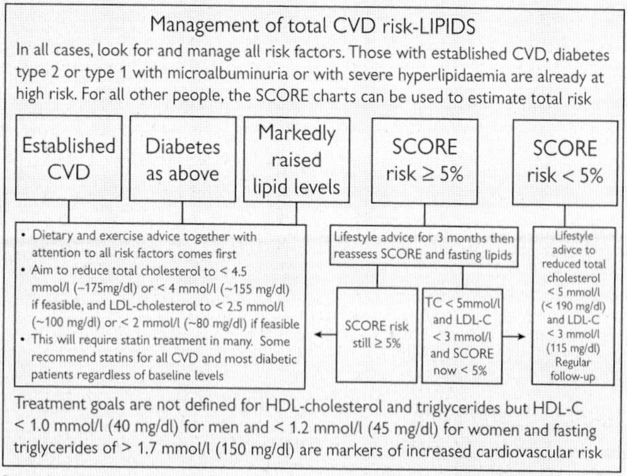
Management of total CVD risk-LIPIDS
In all cases, look for and manage all risk factors. Those with established CVD, diabetes type 2 or type 1 with microalbuminuria or with severe hyperlipidaemia are already at high risk. For all other people, the SCORE charts can be used to estimate total risk
Established CVD
Diabetes as above
Markedly raised lipid levels
SCORE risk ≥ 5%
SCORE risk < 5%
• Dietary and exercise advice together with attention to all risk factors comes first
• Aim to reduce total cholesterol to < 4.5 mmol/l (~175mg/dl) or < 4 mmol/l (~155 mg/dl) if feasible, and LDL-cholesterol to < 2.5 mmol/l (~100 mg/dl) or < 2 mmol/l (~80 mg/dl) if feasible
• This will require statin treatment in many. Some recommend statins for all CVD and most diabetic patients regardless of baseline levels
Lifestyle advice for 3 months then reassess SCORE and fasting lipids
SCORE risk still ≥ 5%
TC < 5mmol/l and LDL-C < 3 mmol/l and SCORE now < 5%
Lifestyle adivce to reduced total cholesterol < 5 mmol/l (< 190 mg/dl) and LDL-C < 3 mmol/l (115 mg/dl) Regular follow-up
Treatment goals are not defined for HDL-cholesterol and triglycerides but HDL-C < 1.0 mmol/l (40 mg/dl) for men and < 1.2 mmol/l (45 mg/dl) for women and fasting triglycerides of > 1.7 mmol/l (150 mg/dl) are markers of increased cardiovascular risk

Reproduced from the original version of the European Guidelines on CVD Prevention. Executive Summary (European Heart Journal 2007;28:2375–2414) and Full text (European journal of Cardiovascular Prevention and Rehabilitation 2007;14(suppl 2): S1-S113). Reproduced with permission of the European Society of Cardiology. © 2007 ESC.

JES4

Lipids targets

- In high risk people, especially those with established CVD or diabetes: total cholesterol < 4.5 mmol/L (~ 175 mg/dL) with an option of < 4.0 mmol/L (~ 155 mg/dL) if feasible; LDL-cholesterol < 2.5 mmol/L (~ 100 mg/dL) with an option of < 2.0 mmol/L (~ 80 mg/dL) if feasible

JBS2

Lipids targets

- In all high risk people the targets for total and LDL cholesterol are < 4 mmol/L (~ 155 mg/dL) or a 25% reduction and < 2 mmol/L (~ 80 mg/dL) or a 25% reduction, respectively

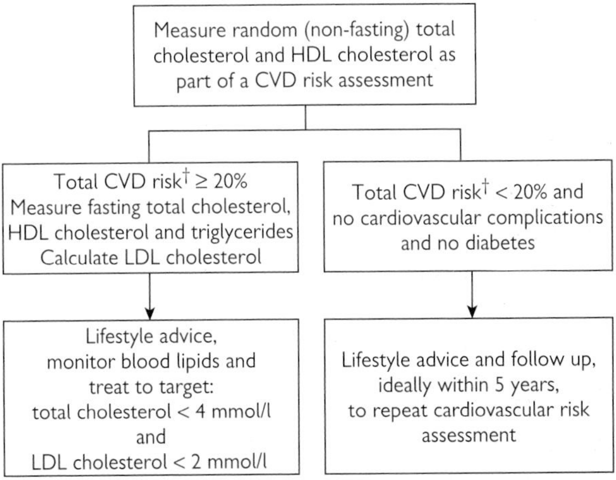

Fig. 10.2 Risk thresholds and targets for blood cholesterol in adsymptomatic people without CVD. †Assessed with CVD risk chart. Reproduced with permission from JBS II British Cardiac Society, British Hypertension Society, Diabetes UK, Primary Care Cardiovascular Society, The Stroke Association. JBS2 (2005) Joint British Societies' guidelines on prevention of cardiovascular disease in clinical practice. *Heart*, 91(Suppl V), V1–V5.

Lipid-lowering drugs

- 3-hydroxy-3-methylglutaryl coenzyme A (HMG-CoA) reductase inhibitors (statins)
- Fibrates
- Bile acid sequestrants (anion exchange resins)
- Niacin or nicotinic acid and its derivates
- Cholesterol absorption inhibitors
- Omega-3 (n-3) fatty acids/ fish oils

Statins

Statins are the corner stone of lipid lowering therapy and have a very strong evidence base for cardiovascular risk reduction in terms of both morbidity and mortality in both primary and secondary prevention.

The decision with regards to which statin is to be used usually depends on cost, local targets and certain patient characteristics (e.g. history of myalgia, renal failure etc).

Whatever statin is used it is important to have some idea of the anticipated LDL-lowering effect. For example, simvastatin 40 mg typically achieves a 38-40 % LDL-lowering effect whilst the more potent statins e.g. atorvastatin 80 mg or rosuvastatin 40 mg typically achieve LDL-lowering in the range of 50-55%.

Remember the 6% Rule

Each doubling of the statin dose produces an average additional decrease in LDL-C levels of only about 5–6%, based upon the baseline LDL-C value. Therefore, if the patient is not achieving target on a certain dose of statin, doubling the dose may only reduce LDL a small amount further. It may be more efficacious to change to a more potent statin.

Combination therapy

If a patient is already on the highest dose of a more potent statin (e.g. atorvastatin 80 mg or rosuvastatin 40 mg) and is still not achieving their lipid targets, and their medication adherence is thought to be good, then combination therapy could be considered. For example, ezetimibe acts independently of statin therapy by blocking intestinal cholesterol absorption. It may further reduce LDL levels by 15-20%.

Niacin, fibrates, bile acid sequestrants and omega-3 fatty acids may also be used in the treatment of dyslipidemia particularly when the triglyceride levels are high or HDL-cholesterol is low, but should be done under advice of a specialist lipid clinic.

Muscle side effects

In clinical practice, muscle side effects are one of the commonest complaints the clinician will have to deal with in patients taking statin therapy.

- Myalgia refers simply to muscle pain (and no weakness) with normal CK levels. Although there is no clear evidence from randomized trials that statins cause myalgia, it is commonly reported. It is important to distinguish the symptoms from other causes of pain such as that from osteoarthritic joints or degenerative back disease.
- Myopathy generally means there is also muscle weakness and accompanied by a rise in creatine kinase levels 10 times the upper limit of normal. Uncommon <0.01% incidence.
- Rhabdomyolysis is severe myopathy and is usually indicated by a CK >40 times the upper limit of normal and renal failure. Very uncommon (less than 1/3 the incidence of myopathy).
- All statins can cause myopathy and rhabdomyolysis, although as a rule of thumb it is usually a dose responsive side effect, i.e. seen with higher doses of statins.

- Other risk factors include renal failure, hypothyroidism, being elderly or concomitant use of drugs that inhibit the cytochrome P450 system (see Box 10.2).
- Combination with the fibrate gemfibrozil should be avoided also due to risk of myopathy, although statins may be used safely with other fibrates (e.g. bezafibrate, fenofibrate). This should be done under specialist supervision.
- In statin myopathy, the statin should be stopped and the patient monitored to ensure that CK levels return to normal. It does not mean that statin therapy is absolutely contraindicated in the future. A less potent statin may be introduced at a low dose, but again this should be done under specialist supervision. Rhabdomyolysis generally requires hospital admission for intravenous fluid therapy. The risk/benefit of the statin should be reviewed.
- Asymptomatic CK levels less than 10 times the upper limit of normal generally do not warrant stopping the statin. It is not advised to routinely measure CK levels.

Box 10.2

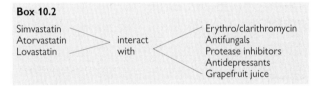

Simvastatin Atorvastatin Lovastatin	interact with	Erythro/clarithromycin Antifungals Protease inhibitors Antidepressants Grapefruit juice

Liver side effects

- A small percentage of patients develop raised transaminases (<1%)
- Higher in intensive statin group
- Generally in first 6 months and the patient is usually asymptomatic
- Usually reversed upon stopping the statin (consider if ALT is >3 times the upper limit of normal)
- Risk of liver failure is probably not above background risk
- Caution in labelling someone as statin intolerant i.e. benefit>risk
- Do measure baseline liver function tests (LFTs)
- Statin product information recommends LFT monitoring when using "higher dose" statins despite lack of evidence on adverse outcome
- Statins are contraindicated in active liver disease. If LFTs are abnormal but stable and there is no active liver disease, it may be reasonable to start statin and monitor

Treatment protocol for glucose management

Classification based on plasma glucose levels

Individuals can be classified into different categories based on fasting plasma glucose and 2-hour plasma glucose levels following a 75 g oral glucose tolerance test (OGTT) (Table 10.2).

Table 10.3 Classification based on plasma glucose levels (reproduced with permission from Graham, I., Atar, D., Borch-Johnsen, K., *et al.* (2007). *European Journal of Cardiovascular Prevention and Rehabilitation*, **14**(Suppl 2), S1–S113)

	Fasting plasma glucose	**2 h plasma glucose**
Normal	≤6.0 mmol/l (≤108 mg/dl)	<7.8 mmol/l (<140 mg/dl)
Impaired fasting glucose[a]	6.1–6.9 mmol/l (110–124 mg/dl)	<7.8 mmol/l (<140 mg/dl)
Impaired glucose tolerance	<7.0 mmol/l (<126 mg/dl)	7.8–11.0 mmol/l (140–198 mg/dl)
Diabetes	≥7.0 mmol/l (≥126 mg/dl)	≥11.1 mmol/l (≥200 mg/dl)

[a] The American Diabetes Association uses ≥5.6 mmol/l (≥100 mg/dl) as the lower cut-off point for impaired fasting glucose. This lower cut-off point was not adapted in Europe, and is not recommended by WHO (© ESC 2007).

Assessment of plasma glucose (JBS2)

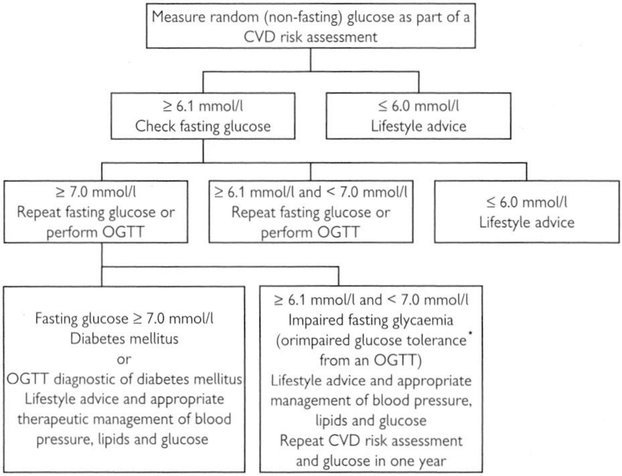

Fig. 10.3 Risk thresholds and targets for plasma blood glucose in asymptomatic people without CVD. *Impaired glucose tolerance: 2-hour glucose in an OGTT ≥7.8 mmol/l and ≤11.0 mmol/l. Reproduced with permission from British Cardiac Society, British Hypertension Society, Diabetes UK, HEART UK, Primary Care Cardiovascular Society, The Stroke Association. JBS2 (2005) Joint British Societies' guidelines on prevention of cardiovascular disease in clinical practice. *Heart*, **91**(Suppl V), V1–V5.

Treatment targets in patients with diabetes

- Fasting plasma glucose <6.0 mmol/l (JES4), ≤6.0 mmol/l (JBS2).
- HbA_{1c} ≤ 6.5%.
- Targets for blood pressure and lipids are as follows.

JES4

- Blood pressure: <130/80 mmHg, if feasible.
- Total cholesterol <4.5 mmol/l (~175 mg/dl) with an option of <4.0 mmol/l (~155 mg/dl) if feasible; LDL cholesterol <2.5 mmol/l (~100 mg/dl) with an option of <2.0 mmol/l (~80 mg/dl) if feasible.

JBS2

- Blood pressure: <130/80 mmHg.
- Total cholesterol <4 mmol/l (~155 mg/dl) or a 25% reduction, and LDL cholesterol <2 mmol/l (~80 mg/dl) or a 25% reduction, respectively.

Management of diabetes

- Patients with diabetes type 2 and type 1 with microalbuminuria are at increased cardiovascular risk.
- Patients with diabetes require multifactorial intervention.
- In type 1 diabetes, glucose control requires appropriate insulin therapy and concomitant professional dietary therapy.
- In type 2 diabetes, professional dietary advice, reduction of overweight, and increased physical activity should be the first treatments. Treatment with oral hypoglycaemic drugs (sulphonylurea, biguanide, thiazolidinediones, or their combination) or insulin may have to be added to the treatment regimen.

Chapter 11

Cardioprotective drug therapies

Antiplatelet therapy

Aspirin

- All with established CVD (including diabetics) unless contraindicated; lifelong treatment with a low dose (75–150 mg daily) is recommended.
- Asymptomatic individuals, aspirin should only be considered when the 10-year risk of CVD mortality is markedly increased and the BP is controlled.

Clopidogrel

- Cases of aspirin allergy.
- In addition to aspirin, in acute coronary syndromes for 9–12 months.
- Combination of aspirin and clopidogrel is not routinely recommended in chronic stable atherosclerotic disease.

Beta-blockers

- Patients post-MI (including diabetics).
- Patients with congestive heart failure (CHF).
- Angina: to relieve the symptoms of myocardial ischaemia.
- As an antihypertensive (other antihypertensives preferred in diabetics).

ACE inhibitors

- Treatment of heart failure or left ventricular dysfunction.
- Diabetics: to reduce BP to target or if type 1 (and possibly type 2) nephropathy.
- To reduce BP to target. Angiotensin receptor blockers can be used in patients with an indication for ACE inhibitors but who cannot tolerate them.

Lipid lowering therapies

- See Chapter 10, p 186-188.

Calcium-channel blockers

- Reducing BP to target.
- Post-MI if beta-blockers are contraindicated.

Diuretics

- Reducing BP to target (alternative antihypertensives are preferred in type 2 diabetes or those at high risk of developing type 2 diabetes).

Anticoagulation

- History of thromboembolic events.
- Left ventricular thrombus.
- Persistent or paroxsymal atrial fibrillation.
- Consider in:
  - large anterior myocardial infarction (MI)
  - left ventricular aneurysm
  - paroxysmal tachyarrythmias (iv) post-MI CHF.

Chapter 12

Erectile dysfunction

Background

Erectile dysfunction (ED) is defined as the inability to attain or maintain penile erections sufficient for satisfactory sexual performance.

It is a common disorder, with an estimated prevalence of ~30–75% of men aged 40–80 years. However, it is thought that nearly 9 out of 10 men with ED do not tell their GP about the problem.

ED may have a significant compromising effect on quality of life and is associated with depression, anxiety, and loss of self-esteem. It is thought that 20% of long-term relationships break down due to erectile dysfunction.

There are multiple aetiological factors, including psychogenic (~25% of cases), physical, or a combination of these (Table 12.1). With pure psychogenic ED, there is usually persistence of nocturnal spontaneous erections.

Non-psychogenic ED is usually due to endothelial dysfunction and atheroma of the penile arteries. Due to the strong association between CVD and its associated risk factors, the recent Second Princeton Consensus on sexual dysfunction and cardiac risk[1] has concluded that a man with ED should be considered at vascular risk until proven otherwise.

Table 12.1 Key factors implicated in ED

Psychogenic	Physical
Stress	Smoking
Fatigue	Sedentary lifestyle
Anxiety and depression	Obesity
Marital dissatisfaction	High alcohol intake
Sexual boredom	High blood pressure
Concerns about sexual orientation	Diabetes
	Medications*
	Lower urinary tract symptoms of benign prostatic hyperplasia
	Testicular failure (rare)

* See Box 12.1

1 Jackson, G., Rosen, R.C., Kloner, R.A., and Kostis, J.B. (2006). The second Princeton consensus on sexual dysfunction and cardiac risk: new guidelines for sexual medicine. *Journal of Sexual Medicine*, **3**(1), 28–36.

Assessment of the patient with ED

A comprehensive assessment should include a sexual medical (including over-the-counter medications), and psychosocial history. Box 12.1 lists the medications implicated in ED.

The IIEF-5 (International Index of Erectile Function) is a standardized and validated questionnaire which may be used for consistency in diagnosis and grading of the severity of ED, with a score of 5–7 indicating severe ED.

Examination

A focused physical exam including that of the cardiovascular system, genitalia, and digital rectal examination should be performed. Evidence of loss of secondary sexual characteristics (indicative of testicular failure) should be sought.

Investigations

The history and physical examination should generally guide further investigations and if the ED is thought to be organic, a full blood count, blood glucose, lipid profile, urea and creatinine, and, in some cases, testosterone levels may be warranted. If a local or hormonal cause is suspected, then referral to urology services should be considered.

Box 12.1 Medications implicated in ED

Diuretics, e.g. thiazides, spironolactone
Antihypertensives, e.g. beta-blockers, calcium-channel blockers
Lipid-lowering, e.g. clofibrate
Antidepressants, e.g. selective serotonin reuptake inhibitors (SSRIs)
H_2 antagonists, e.g. ranitidine
Hormones, e.g. 5-alpha-reductase inhibitors
Recreational drugs, e.g. cocaine, alcohol

Management

There is some evidence that weight loss, exercise, and smoking cessation may improve erectile function.

For those with non-organic ED, sex counselling/couple therapy could be considered.

Phosphodiesterase type 5 (PDE-5) inhibitors

These oral agents are the mainstay of therapy and act by increasing levels of cyclic guanosine monophosphate (GMP) which helps relax smooth muscle cells and increase blood flow in the penis. N.B. Foreplay/sexual stimulation is still required.

Three PDE-5 inhibitors—sildenafil, vardenafil, and tadalafil—are currently available. The main difference between them is that sildenafil and vardenafil have a shorter half-life (~4 hours) than tadalafil (~17.5 hours).

- Patients should be started on a middle dose of chosen medication, then titrated until a response is achieved.
- Success rates of 65–75% are reported but are least successful in those with diabetes, likely due to concomitant neural involvement.
- If unsuccessful after the highest dose on six different occasions, try an alternative PDE-5 inhibitor.
- The medication should not be used more than once in 24 hours.
- Main side-effects include headache, facial flushing, rhinitis, and dyspepsia.

PDE-5 inhibitors in patients with cardiovascular disease

Generally these drugs have similar favourable safety profiles with no adverse haemodynamic effects and no increased incidence of myocardial infarction. However, a patient's cardiovascular status should be evaluated prior to starting treatment.

Princeton guidelines for the treatment of erectile dysfunction in men with coronary artery disease

Table 12.2 Princeton guidelines

Risk level	Recommendation
Low: asymptomatic coronary artery disease and fewer than three of the following risk factors: controlled hypertension, mild stable angina, successful coronary revascularization, previous uncomplicated myocardial infarction, mild valvular disease, and congestive heart failure (left ventricular dysfunction with or without NYHA Class I)	Possible use of PDE-5 inhibitor
Coronary artery disease and fewer than three of the following risk factors: moderate angina, myocardial infarction (>2 but <6 weeks), left ventricular dysfunction, or congestive heart failure (NYHA Class II)	Further evaluation by a cardiologist
Unstable angina, uncontrolled hypertension, congestive heart failure (Class III–IV), recent myocardial infarction (<2 weeks), high-risk arrythmias, hypertrophic obstructive or other cardiomyopathy, and moderate to severe valvular heart disease	No treatment until condition stabilized

Note

A major contraindication (CI) is concomitant nitrate use including GTN® spray (dual vasodilation leads to a profound hypotensive effect). Past use of nitrates more than 2 weeks previously is not considered a CI.

- If patients develop angina during sexual intercourse, they should be advised to rest for 5–10 min, and if pain persists >15 min, to seek emergency care.
- Advised not to take nitrates for 24 hours after sildenafil and vardenafil, and for 48 hours after tadalafil (due to its longer half-life).
- PDE-s inhibitors should not be used in conjunction with nicorandil due to possible risk of hypotension.
- Vardenafil is not recommended in patients who take Class Ia/3 anti-arrythmics or in those with congenitally prolonged QTc.
- Caution with the use of alpha-blockers.

Other therapies

Other therapeutic options include:

- Prostaglandin therapy through either intracavernous injection or intra-urethral pessary.
- Mechanical—vacuum pump or rigid penile implants.
- Hormonal therapy.

These services are usually available in specialist units.

Key references

McVary, T. (2008). Erectile dysfunction. *New England Journal of Medicine*, **357**, 2472–81.

Watts, G.F., Chew, K.K., and Stuckey, B.G. (2007). The erectile-endothelial dysfunction nexus: new opportunities for cardiovascular risk prevention. *Nature Clinical Practice Cardiovascular Medicine*, **4**(5), 263-–3.

Chapter 13

The health promotion workshop programme

The health promotion workshop group

Group health promotion workshops provide an important learning opportunity. Health promotion comprises a key aspect in the role of all members of the team. They must assess and understand the illness perceptions, health beliefs, and risk perception of patients and their families if they are to empower patients and families to make healthy choices.

Aim of the workshops

- To empower patients and families with the genuine potential to make choices.
- To raise critical awareness of the issues relating to their health.
- To develop a high level of realistic self-esteem and life skills.

Knowledge empowers patients and their families to become involved in their own healthcare and may influence the sustaining of lifestyle changes, adherence to medication regimens, coping and social and emotional adaptation, and recovery.

Who should facilitate the workshops?

A member of the programme team or other professional who has specialist knowledge of the subject. For example, the workshop on cardioprotective medications may be best delivered by a pharmacist, and the workshop on the benefits of physical activity would be best delivered by the physiotherapist/physical activity specialist.

Programme

The workshops should:

- Provide information
- Be interactive
- Encourage questions and discussion
- Clarify goals
- Identify and correct misconceptions.

A rolling programme of eight workshops is recommended, which covers the topics outlined in Table 13.1.

Table 13.1 Proposed programme for health promotion workshops

No.	Workshop details	Delivered by
1	Understanding cardiovascular disease management and prevention: focus on cholesterol	Nurse and dietitian
2	Reducing risk factors for cardiovascular disease: focus on smoking, blood pressure, and diabetes/glucose	Nurse
3	Lifestyle risks and cardiovascular disease: healthy eating—choosing the right foods	Dietitian
4	Understanding cardioprotective medications	Pharmacist, nurse, or doctor
5	Stress management and relaxation	Nurse, occupational therapist
6	Lifestyle risks and cardiovascular disease: the benefits of exercise	Physical activity specialist
7	Food labelling and weight management	Dietitian
8	Maintaining lifestyle changes	Nurse
Optional	Supermarket visit	Dietitian
For smokers	Smokers' workshop	Nurse

Learning outcomes of the workshops

Understanding cardiovascular disease and risk factors: focus on cholesterol

Aim: To educate patients and their families about CVD; what it is, the risk factors, and how it is managed.

At the end of the session each of the participants will be able to:
- Explain how the heart and arteries work.
- Explain the process of atherosclerosis and how it can lead to coronary heart disease, stroke, peripheral vascular disease, and renal disease.
- Explain the management of CVD.
- Explain what action to take in the event of an angina attack.
- Identify the risk factors for heart disease.
- Explain what cholesterol is, what affects it, and what the target should be.

Understanding cardiovascular disease and risk factors: focus on blood pressure, diabetes, and smoking

Aim: To educate families about the risk factors for CVD.

At the end of the session each of the participants will be able to:
- List the risk factors for heart disease and understand the concept of total risk.
- Explain what blood pressure is, what affects it, and what their target should be.
- Explain what diabetes is, what affects it, and related targets.
- Understand the degree of risk that smoking contributes to total CVD, list smoking cessation methods, and be aware of support networks.

Healthy eating—choosing the right foods

Aim: To encourage families to follow a healthy eating pattern that is in line with the current heart health guidelines for heart disease.

At the end of the session each of the participants will be able to:
- List the key messages for diet and prevention of CVD.
- Identify other dietary factors that can affect CVD.

Understanding cardioprotective medications

Aim: To educate patients and families about the action of prescribed cardioprotective medications and to encourage compliance.

At the end of the session each of the participants will be able to:
- Understand the prescribed medication, including mode of action, and the common side-effects.
- Recognize the importance of taking medication regularly, and that medication may have to be taken throughout life.

Stress management

Aim: To educate patients and families about stress management.

At the end of the session each of the participants will be able to:
- Explain what stress is.
- Identify positive and negative aspects of stress.
- Identify what are their symptoms of stress are.
- Identify barriers they can build up to reduce stressful situations.

Weight management and food labelling

Aim: To encourage families to maintain or improve their weight and shape, to reduce their risk of CVD, and to have an understanding of the labelling of food products.

At the end of the session each of the participants will be able to:

- List the health risks of obesity.
- Identify what is a healthy weight and shape, including suitable target levels for themselves.
- Identify possible weight loss strategies.
- Identify nutritional claims that are on products that they buy, and have an understanding of what they mean.
- Choose the healthier product from the nutritional information supplied on the selected products.

Maintaining change

Aim: To encourage families to maintain any lifestyle changes they have made and help them to identify strategies to maintain these changes.

At the end of the session each of the participants will be able to:

- Understand the process of behaviour change.
- Identify strategies to help them maintain changes they have made.
- Identify personal ways of motivation to maintain changes, including planning next goals.
- Identify way of coping with, and planning to avoid, relapse.

The benefits of exercise

Aim: The aim of this session is to help patients and families to understand the benefits and current recommendations around physical activity and exercise in the prevention of CVD and to empower individuals with the knowledge and confidence to participate in safe and effective levels of physical activity.

At the end of this session the participants will be able to:

- List the health benefits associated with physical activity.
- Identify some of the more common barriers to participation.
- State the frequency, intensity, duration, and types of activities associated with the most health benefit in terms of prevention of CVD.
- Identify key exercise precautions and activities that should be avoided.

Note

It is important to acknowledge that many in the group may be very active, while others may not. The purpose of this talk is not to 'preach' about exercise but more to outline the recommendations of what type of exercise is the most effective, as many people underdo physical activity while others overdo it in response to a cardiac event or being identified at high cardiovascular risk. The session tries to stimulate everyone to feel they could do something realistic to increase and maintain physical activity safely as part of their everyday living.

Characteristics of the workshop facilitator

- ***Teaching ability:*** knowledge of the subject, ability to communicate, managing groups of adults with mixed ability.
- ***Manner:*** acceptance by participants, non-judgemental attitude, friendliness, not patronizing.
- ***Recognition:*** draws on the wealth of knowledge and experience of the participants.
- ***Raises critical awareness:*** facilitates the formation of new insights from existing and new knowledge, encourages self-direction.
- ***Relevance:*** ensures that the workshop is culturally sensitive to the participants (for example, food choices with ethnic minorities) and relevant to their learning needs (talking about smoking to a group where the majority do not smoke).

Teaching methods

Box 13.1 Some ideas for teaching adults

- Make the workshops interactive and invite active contribution from participants.
- Use mini quizzes and tasks. They can be fun and help learning at the same time.
- Repeat and reinforce information throughout the programme.
- Divide participants into small work groups during workshops, to encourage interaction, and then bring them together at the end, to encourage feedback and discussion.
- Group discussion allows participants to explore the information given and how best to apply it to themselves and their families. The sessions should be informal and encourage participants to recognize their own risk factors and develop strategies for change.
- Assess knowledge by eliciting contributions and writing them on a flip chart.
- The following resources are useful:
  - heart model
  - flip charts and pens
  - PowerPoint
  - electronic risk calculator (HEARTSCORE, JBS2)
  - empty food packages to explain food labelling.
- Practice relaxation techniques.
- Role play.

Chapter 14

Data management, quality assurance, and audit

The data collected on each participant should be recorded and stored on a dedicated secure database.

Clinical activity

A secure database is important for:

- Recruitment monitoring.
- Tracking of changes in clinical measurements, e.g. blood pressure/ weight/medications.
- Automated generation of letters for communication with patient's general practitioner and others.

Data quality

A secure database is important to:

- Promote recording of data in a consistent and standardized manner.
- Enable internal validation measures to promote accuracy of the data collected.
- Facilitate elimination of missing data.

Audit

Audit of the programme's outcomes according to recognized guidelines (e.g. JBS2[1]) and treatment protocols is important for evaluating both the clinical effectiveness of the programme and the quality of care provided. In addition, contribution to either regional or national datasets (e.g. the UK National Audit of Cardiac Rehabilitation[2]) is important for informing service delivery needs. A European cardiac rehabilitation data set (CARDS system[3]) is also being developed.

1 JBS2 (2006). Joint British Societies' guidelines on prevention of cardiovascular disease in clinical practice. *Heart*, **91**(Suppl V), 1–52.

2 http://www.cardiacrehabilitation.org.uk/dataset.htmNACR

3 http://www.escardio.org/knowledge/ehs/registries/cards.htm

Index

N

O

P